Managing Gastrointestinal Complications of Diabetes

Joseph Sellin
Editor

Managing Gastrointestinal Complications of Diabetes

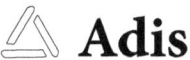

Editor
Joseph Sellin
Baylor College of Medicine
Houston, Texas, USA

ISBN 978-3-319-48661-1   ISBN 978-3-319-48662-8   (eBook)
DOI 10.1007/978-3-319-48662-8

Library of Congress Control Number: 2016963589

Printed on acid-free paper

This Adis imprint is published by Springer Nature
The registered company is Springer International Publishing AG
The registered company address is Gewerbestrasse 11, 6330 Cham, Switzerland

Editor Biography

Professor Joseph Sellin, MD, graduated from Amherst College and Albert Einstein College of Medicine. He did his Internal Medicine Training at Montefiore Medical Center and Gastroenterology Fellowship at the University of Chicago and spent a sabbatical at Stanford University. Professor Sellin joined the faculty at the University of Texas Medical School in 1980 and was Division Director and Fellowship Director from 1990 to 2002. From 2003 to 2009, he was Professor of Medicine, Director of the GI Fellowship, and Director of the IBD Center at UTMB–Galveston. Since 2009, Dr. Sellin has served as Chief of Gastroenterology at Ben Taub Hospital, Director of the GI Fellowship, and Professor of Medicine at Baylor College of Medicine. His research interests have focused on intestinal fluid and electrolyte transport, chronic diarrhea, and inflammatory bowel disease. He has held leadership positions in the American Gastroenterological Association, the American College of Gastroenterology, and the Crohn's and Colitis Foundation of America. He is the author of more than 100 manuscripts and book chapters. Dr. Sellin is a member of Phi Beta Kappa and the American Society for Clinical Investigation.

Contents

Chapter 1
Introduction

Ruchi Gaba

1.1 Introduction

Diabetes mellitus (DM) is one of the most prevalent chronic diseases in the world. As of 2013, 382 million people had diabetes, and it has been estimated that this number will reach 592 million in 2035, making DM a major public health problem worldwide [1]. With improvements in therapies, survival has increased and majority of the patients now live with long-term complications of the disease. Gastrointestinal (GI) symptoms occur more commonly in patients with diabetes than in the general population [2]. In fact, GI symptoms such as nausea, abdominal pain, bloating, diarrhea, constipation, and delayed gastric emptying occur in almost 75 % of patients with diabetes [3]. A majority of patients with GI symptoms stay undiagnosed or undertreated due to a lack of awareness of these complications among clinicians. In order to improve care and health-related quality of life in these patients, a high index of suspicion, early identification, and appropriate management of GI complications are mandatory.

R. Gaba
Endocrinology, Diabetes and Metabolism,
Baylor College of Medicine, Houston, TX, USA
e-mail: ruchi.gaba@bcm.edu

J. Sellin (ed.), *Managing Gastrointestinal Complications of Diabetes*, DOI 10.1007/978-3-319-48662-8_1,
© Springer International Publishing AG 2017

Diabetes can affect the entire GI tract from the oral cavity and esophagus to the large bowel and anorectal region, either in isolation or in a combination. The extent and the severity of the presenting symptoms may vary widely depending upon which part of the GI tract is involved. In patients with long-term type 1 DM, upper GI symptoms seem to be particularly common [4]. Of the different types (Fig. 1.1), including esophageal dysmotility, gastroesophageal reflux disease (GERD), diabetic diarrhea, constipation, enteropathy, and nonalcoholic fatty liver disease (NAFLD), gastroparesis seems to be the most well known and most serious complication, occurring in about 50 % of patients with diabetes-related GI complications [5].

1.2   Risk Factors

Elevated blood glucose (HbA1c), long duration of diabetes, and the presence of established macro- and microvascular complications are some of the risk factors associated with

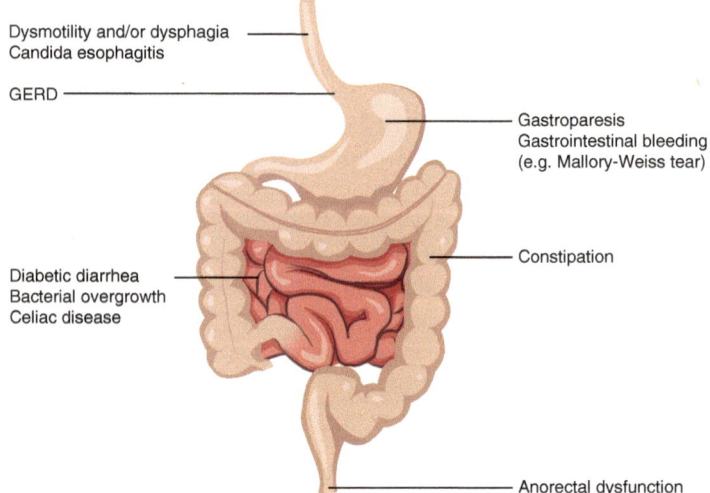

FIGURE 1.1 Gastrointestinal complications associated with diabetes (Reproduced with permission from Sellin [11] ©Nature)

development of gastroparesis [6]. Women have been found to have a higher risk of developing these complications than men [4]. This can be partly explained by the fact that females in general tend to have higher rates of GI symptoms and functional disorders irrespective of whether they have diabetes [7]. They also tend to seek health care more frequently than the men. Female patients with diabetes, in particular, have an increased incidence of eating disturbances [8]. The GI transit time is significantly prolonged during the luteal phase of the menstrual cycle when progesterone levels are increased compared with the follicular phase [9]. However, the exact role of ovarian hormones on gastric emptying is still unclear [10].

1.3 Etiology and Clinical Presentation

The enteric nervous system (ENS) is an independent network of neurons and glial cells that spread from the esophagus up to the internal anal sphincter. Structured as two major plexuses, myenteric (Auerbach's) and the submucous (Meissner's) plexus, the ENS regulates GI tract functions including motility, secretion, and participation in immune regulation [12, 13]. GI complications and their symptoms in patients with diabetes arise secondary to both abnormalities of gastric function (sensory and motor modality), as well as impairment of GI hormonal secretion [14], but these abnormalities are complex and incompletely understood. Over the last several years, knowledge of the mechanisms of DM-induced changes in GI tract has expanded. It has been known for a long time that diabetic autonomic neuropathy (i.e., dysfunction of the neurons supplying the ENS) leads to abnormalities in the GI motility, sensation, secretion, and absorption, serving as the main pathogenic mechanism underlying GI complications.

Recently, evidence has emerged to suggest that other processes might also play a role. Loss of the pacemaker interstitial cells of Cajal, impairment of the inhibitory nitric oxide-containing nerves, abnormal myenteric neurotransmission, smooth muscle dysfunction, and imbalances in the number of excitatory and inhibitory enteric neurons can drastically alter complex motor functions causing dysfunction of the enteric system [7, 11, 15, 16]. This dysfunction can further lead to the development of dysphagia and reflux esophagitis in the esophagus, gastroparesis, and dyspepsia in the stomach, pseudo-obstruction of the small intestine, and constipation, diarrhea, and incontinence in the colon.

In animal models of DM (i.e., streptozocin-induced DM in rats), defective tropic signaling of neurotransmitters (vasoactive intestinal peptide, acetylcholine, substance P, nucleotides), paracrine agents (serotonin), anti-inflammatory agents (prostaglandins, leukotrienes), histamine, and loss of adrenergic enteric innervation can also cause abnormalities in epithelial function and development, resulting in enhanced nutrient transport and abnormalities in salt and water transport [17, 18]. Compromised intestinal vascular flow arising due to ischemia and hypoxia from microvascular disease of the GI tract can also cause abdominal pain, bleeding, and mucosal dysfunction.

Mitochondrial dysfunction has been implicated in the pathogenesis of gastric neuropathy. It involves the degeneration of dorsal root ganglion neurons in peripheral nerves; dorsal root ganglion mitochondria are particularly effected [19]. Formation of irreversible advanced glycation end products (AGE) can cause qualitative and quantitative changes in extracellular matrix components such as type IV collagen, laminin, and vitronectin. This can affect cell adhesion, growth, and matrix accumulation. AGE-modified proteins also alter cell function by interacting with specific receptors on macrophages and endothelial cells, inducing changes that promote matrix overproduction, focal thrombosis, and vasoconstriction [20].

Motility alterations can cause overgrowth of the small bowel microflora and induce bloating, diarrhea, abdominal pain, and malabsorption [21]. However, there is some evidence to suggest that the diarrhea might actually be due to colonic bacterial metabolism of carbohydrate secondary to rapid small bowel transit rather than small bowel bacterial overgrowth [22].

Acute and chronic hyperglycemia or hypoglycemia which can alter intestinal function by affecting the metabolic and signaling pathway of the enteric neurons and effect gut motility [16, 23–26]. Acute (insulin induced) hypoglycemia accelerates gastric emptying [27]. Thus GI motor function is highly sensitive to fluctuations in glycemic state. Hyperglycemia can also cause vagal inhibition leading to acute GI symptoms [15]. Another possible association between DM and the gastrointestinal tract can be infrequent autoimmune diseases associated with type I DM like autoimmune chronic pancreatitis, celiac disease (2–11 %), and autoimmune gastropathy (2 % prevalence in general population and three- to fivefold increase in patients with typc 1 DM) [28, 29].

GI symptoms are often associated with the presence of other diabetic complications, especially autonomic and peripheral neuropathy [2, 30, 31]. In fact, patients with microvascular complications such as retinopathy, nephropathy, or neuropathy should be presumed to have GI abnormalities until proven otherwise. In a large cross-sectional questionnaire study of 1,101 subjects with DM, 57 % of patients reported at least one GI complication [31]. Poor glycemic control has also been found to be associated with increased severity of the upper GI symptoms. There is some discordant data linking diabetic autonomic neuropathy to the duration of diabetes, but the Diabetes Control and Complications Trial suggested that, at least in persons with type 1 DM, neuropathy and other GI complications are associated with poor glycemic control, rather than the duration of diabetes [32].

1.4   Diagnosis

Establishing a diagnosis of GI autonomic neuropathy is difficult as there are no tests available to evaluate the GI innervation and autonomic tone directly. Moreover, the cardiovascular alterations are of low value in the prediction of motor alterations of the GI tract. The most widely available and standard method for evaluating motility disorders and assessing gastric emptying is scintigraphy. Other alternatives include radiolabeled breath testing and wireless motility capsule testing [33, 34]. Techniques such as ultrasound, single-photon emission computed tomography (SPECT), and magnetic resonance imaging (MRI) are predominantly research tools used for evaluating gastric volume, contractility, distribution of meals, and emptying.

1.5   Treatment Options

The fundamental basis of treating gastroparesis is dietary modification, such as eating frequent, small, soft meals with a low fat or fiber content. Beyond dietary changes, the management of gastroparesis includes Food and Drug Administration (FDA)-approved D2 receptor antagonists and 5-HT4 agonist metoclopramide, the long-term use of which is limited by side effects such as restlessness and acute dystonia, including tardive dyskinesia. Another alternative is domperidone, a D2-receptor antagonist, which does not carry the same risk of extrapyramidal side effects, but is it not FDA approved and is not marketed for sale in Europe or the United States. In addition, erythromycin, a prokinetic drug which is administered either orally or parenterally, can improve gastric emptying time and reduce nausea and vomiting by its molecular mimicking of motilin. For refractory cases of gastroparesis, gastric electrical stimulation with endoscopically implanted electrodes has been in use since its approval by FDA in 2000 [35].

Lately, muscarinic receptor antagonists and 5HT4-, D2-, ghrelin, and motilin receptor agonists (without antibiotic action) are being evaluated as newer therapeutic agents to control symptoms due to gastroparesis [36, 37]. Diarrhea secondary to diabetic visceral neuropathy can be a troubling GI complication and has been shown to be treated effectively and safely with loperamide. Constipation can be relieved by laxative use, but in recent years, agents such as lubiprostone have been used to relieve constipation not adequately treated by laxatives. Another newer therapeutic approach for treating constipation is stimulation of epithelial guanylate cyclase-C (GC-C) receptor on intestinal epithelial cells [37]. Linaclotide is approved for treatment of constipation and acts by binding to this specific receptor; it is used with spare use of opiate agents for the same reason. Patients with neuropathy also suffering from chronic abdominal pain may respond to agents such as low-dose tricyclic antidepressants (TCAs), selective serotonin reuptake inhibitors (SSRIs), and selective serotonin-noradrenaline reuptake inhibitors (SNRIs). It helps reduce opiate agents for the same reason.

GI symptoms are also commonly reported as side effects of oral hypoglycemic agents particularly metformin and alpha-glucosidase inhibitors. However it is hard to prove a causal relationship as it is difficult to distinguish between spontaneous and true drug-related symptoms due to the high incidence of background GI symptoms in these patients. The most frequent symptoms caused by these medications include diarrhea and vomiting, which can lead to poorer quality of life and reduced compliance with treatment. Newer agents targeting the incretin system like glucagon-like peptide (GLP)-1 receptor agonists and dipeptidyl peptidase 4 (DPP-4) inhibitors are increasingly being used to treat type 2 diabetes. GLP-1 agonists increase insulin secretion while inhibiting glucagon release. They also delay gastric emptying and help decrease food intake. Their most common adverse effect includes mild to moderate GI symptoms particularly nausea, vomiting, and diarrhea. But the nausea tends to be transient and can be reduced with dose titration (Table 1.1). Acute pancreatitis has been associated with DPP-4 inhibitors use but causal relationship has not been established [38]. Liver function test needs to be monitored with certain DPP4-inhibitors such as vildagliptin and alogliptin [39].

As noted in various epidemiological studies, type 2 DM is associated with a significantly increased risk of colorectal, pancreatic, and hepatic cancer [40–42]; few studies have explored links with type 1. Type 2 DM is also associated with an increase in cancer mortality, especially colorectal cancer [40, 43]. There is insufficient evidence that antihyperglycemic

TABLE 1.1 Antihyperglycemic medications and their gastrointestinal (GI)-related side effects

Antihyperglycemic medications	GI-related side effects
Biguanides	Dyspepsia, nausea, abdominal cramping, and diarrhea
Metformin	Risk of lactic acidosis
Sulfonylureas (second generation)	Weight gain
Glipizide	
Glimepiride	
Gliclazide	
Glyburide/glibenclamide	
Thiazolidinediones	Weight gain and fluid retention
Pioglitazone	
Rosiglitazone	
Alpha-glucosidase inhibitors	Bloating, diarrhea, and flatulence
Acarbose	Elevated transaminases
Miglitol	
GLP-1 agonist	Nausea, vomiting, diarrhea
Exenatide	Sense of fullness, early satiety? Increased risk of pancreatitis
Liraglutide	
Lixisenatide	
Dulaglutide	
Albiglutide	

TABLE 1.1 (continued)

Antihyperglycemic medications	GI-related side effects
DDP-4 inhibitors	Diarrhea and abdominal discomfort? Increased risk of pancreatitis
Saxagliptin	
Linagliptin	
Sitagliptin	
Alogliptin	
Dopamine 2- agonist	Nausea
Bromocriptine	
Amylin mimetic	Nausea, vomiting
Pramlintide	Enhances satiety
Bile acid sequestrant	GI intolerance, constipation
Colesevelam	
Meglitinides	Weight gain
Repaglinide	
Nateglinide	
SGLT2 inhibitors	GI neutral
Canagliflozin	
Dapagliflozin	
Empagliflozin	

agents are definitively associated with an increased cancer risk, though available epidemiological data supports an association with metformin and a neutral-to-decreased effect on cancer incidence and mortality [44]. While diabetes and cancer share hormonal imbalances such as increased insulin/ IGF-1 (insulin-like growth factor-1) or leptin/adiponectin secretion, immune abnormalities including elevated circulating pro-inflammatory cytokines, and metabolic alterations (linked to obesity), the exact underlying biological mechanisms linking these two diseases are not completely understood.

Hyperinsulinemia can affect cancer development in many complex ways. In cancer cells, the insulin receptor (IR) is overexpressed and the A isoform (with insulin-mediated mitogenic effect) is overexpressed in comparison to B isoform. The A isoform can stimulate insulin-mediated mitogenesis, even in cells deficient in IGF-1 receptors. Insulin can bind and activate IGF-1 receptors (more potent mitogenic and antiapoptotic activity than IR). In addition, insulin can reduce hepatic production of IGF-binding proteins and further increase free-circulating IGF-1 [45]. Moreover, the mitogenic effect of insulin might be enhanced by post-receptor molecular mechanisms [46, 47] as well. In regard to hyperglycemia and its role in cancer development, there has been a recent resurgence of "Warburg effect" and its relation to cancer energetics [48], where tumor cells appear to use glycolysis for generating ATP instead of oxidative phosphorylation. This requires much more glucose, creating an environment of excess glucose in tumor cells. Glucose is one source of energy, but tumor cells can derive energy from other sources such as glutamine and transform intracellular signaling and adjust metabolic pathways to proliferate [49].

Hence, management of DM-induced GI complications is challenging, is generally suboptimal, and needs improvement. With our increased understanding of the GI complications of diabetes, an integrative approach with better glycemic control and amelioration of the symptomatic manifestations of GI complications should be followed for better care. In Chap. 2, the pathophysiology and treatment of the various common GI complications will be reviewed in more detail.

References

1. Guariguata L, Whiting DR, Hambleton I, Beagley J, Linnenkamp U, Shaw JE. Global estimates of diabetes prevalence for 2013 and projections for 2035. Diabetes Res Clin Pract. 2014;103:137–49.

2. Bytzer P, Talley NJ, Leemon M, Young LJ, Jones MP, Horowitz M. Prevalence of gastrointestinal symptoms associated with diabetes mellitus: a population-based survey of 15,000 adults. Arch Intern Med. 2001;161:1989–96.

3. Feldman M, Schiller LR. Disorders of GI motility associated with diabetes mellitus. Ann Intern Med. 1983;98:378–84.

4. Schvarcz E, Palmér M, Ingberg CM, Aman J, Berne C. Increased prevalence of upper gastrointestinal symptoms in long-term type 1 diabetes mellitus. Diabet Med. 1996;13:478.

5. Smith D, Williams C, Ferris C. Diagnosis and treatment of chronic gastroparesis and chronic intestinal pseudo-obstruction. Gastroenterol Clin N Am. 2003;32:619–58.

6. Camilleri M. Diabetic gastroparesis. N Engl J Med. 2007;356:820–82.

7. Talley NJ et al. Systemic review: the prevalence and clinical course of functional dyspepsia. Aliment Pharmacol Ther. 2004;19:643–54.

8. Rosmark B, Berne C, Holmgren S, Lago C, Renholm G, Sohlberg S. Eating disorders in patients with insulin-dependent diabetes. J Clin Psychiatry. 1986;16:49–57.

9. Gill RC, Murphy PD, Hooper HR, Bowes KL, Kingma YJ. Effect of menstrual cycle on gastric emptying. Digestion. 1987;36:168–74.

10. Wald A, Van Thiel DH, Hoechstetter L, Gavaler JS, Egler KM, Verm R, Scott L, Lester R. Gastrointestinal transit: the effect of the menstrual cycle. Gastroenterology. 1981;80:1497–500.

11. Sellin JH, Chang EB. Therapy insight: gastrointestinal complications of diabetes—pathophysiology and management. Nature. 2008;5:162–71.

12. Costa M, Brookes SJ. The enteric nervous system. Am J Gastroenterol. 1994;89:S129–37.

13. Goyal RK, Hirano I. The enteric nervous system. N Engl J Med. 1996;334:1106–15.

14. Ziegler D. Diagnosis and treatment of diabetic autonomic neuropathy. Curr Diabetes Rep. 2001;1:216–27.

15. Takahashi T, Matsuda K, Kono T, Pappas TN. Inhibitory effects of hyperglycemia on neural activity of the vagus in rats. Intensive Care Med. 2003;29:309–11.

16. He CL, Soffer EE, Ferris CD, Walsh RM, Szurszewski JH, Farrugia G. Loss of interstitial cells of Cajal and inhibitory innervation in insulin-dependent diabetes. Gastroenterology. 2001;121:427–34.

17. Fedorak RN. Intestinal adaptation to diabetes. Altered Na-dependent nutrient absorption in streptozocin-treated chronically diabetic rats. J Clin Invest. 1987;79:1571–8.
18. Chang EB, Bergenstal RM, Field M. Diarrhea in streptozocin treated rats. Loss of adrenergic regulation of intestinal fluid and electrolyte transport. J Clin Invest. 1985;75:1666–70.
19. Leinninger GM, Edwards JL, Lipshaw MJ, Feldman EL. Mechanism of disease: mitochondria as new therapeutic target in diabetic neuropathy. Nat Clin Pract Neurol. 2006;2:620–8.
20. Brownlee M. Glycation products and the pathogenesis of diabetic complications. Diabetes Care. 1992;15:1835–43.
21. Kopacova M. Small intestinal bacterial overgrowth syndrome. World J Gastroenterol. 2010;16:2978–90.
22. Sellin JH, Hart R. Glucose malabsorption associated with rapid intestinal transit. Am J Gastroenterol. 1992;87:584–9.
23. Fedorak RN, Field M, Chang EB. Treatment of diabetic diarrhea with clonidine. Ann Intern Med. 1985;102:197–9.
24. Lacy BE, Crowell MD, Schettler-Duncan A, Mathis C, Pasricha PJ. The treatment of diabetic gastroparesis with botulinum toxin injection into the pylorus. Diabetes Care. 2004;27:2341–7.
25. Rabine JC, Barnett JL. Management of the patient with gastroparesis. J Clin Gastroenterol. 2001;32:11–21.
26. Takahara H, Fujimura M, Taniguchi S, Hayashi N, Nakamura T, Fujimiya M. Changes in serotonin levels and 5-HT receptor activity in duodenum of streptozotocin-diabetic rats. Am J Physiol Gastrointest Liver Physiol. 2001;281:G798–808.
27. Russo A, Stevens J, Chen R, Gentilcore D, Burnet R, Horowitz M, et al. Insulin- induced hypoglycemia accelerates gastric emptying of solids and liquids in long standing type 1 diabetes. J Clin Endocrinol Metab. 2005;90:4489–95.
28. De Block CE, De Leeuw IH, Van Gaal LF. High prevalence of manifestations of gastric autoimmunity in parietal cell antibody-positive type 1 (insulin- dependent) diabetic patients. The Belgian Diabetes Registry. J Clin Endocrinol Metab. 1999;84:4062–7.
29. Aggarwal S, Lebwohl B, Green PHR. Screening for celiac disease in average- risk and high – risk populations. Ther Adv Gastroenterol. 2012;5:37–47.
30. The Diabetes Control and Complications Trial Research Group. The effect of intensive treatment of diabetes on the development and progression of long-term complications in insulin-dependent diabetes mellitus. N Engl J Med. 1993;329:977–86.

31. Bytzer P, Talley NJ, Hammer J, Young LJ, Jones MP, Horowitz M. GI symptoms in diabetes mellitus are associated with both poor glycemic control and diabetic complications. Am J Gastroenterol. 2002;97:604–11.
32. Diabetes Control and Complications Trial Research Group. The effect of intensive treatment of diabetes on the development and progression of long term complications in insulin dependent diabetes mellitus. N Engl J Med. 1993;329:977–86.
33. Timm D, Willis H, Thomas W, Sanders L, Boileau T, Slavin J. The use of a wireless motility device (SmartPill) for the measurement of gastrointestinal transit time after a dietary fiber intervention. Br J Nutr. 2011;105:1337–42.
34. Sarosiek I, Selover KH, Katz LA, Semler JR, Wilding GE, Lackner JM, et al. The assessment of regional gut transit times in healthy controls and patients with gastroparesis using wireless motility technology. Aliment Pharmacol Ther. 2010;31:313–22.
35. Chu H, Lin Z, Zhong L, McCallum RW, Hou X. Treatment of high-frequency gastric electrical stimulation for gastroparesis. J Gastroenterol Hepatol. 2012;27:1017–26.
36. Horvath VJ, Vittal H, Lörincz A, Chen H, Almeida-Porada G, Redelman D, et al. Reduced stem cell factor links smooth myopathy and loss of interstitial cells of Cajal in murine diabetic gastroparesis. Gastroenterology. 2006;130:759–70.
37. AJ L, CB K, JE M, BJ L, MG C, DA F, et al. Efficacy of linaclotide for patients with chronic constipation. Gastroenterology. 2010;138:886–95.
38. L L, Shen J, MM B, JW B, Ebrahim S, PO V. Incretin treatment and risk of pancreatitis in patients with type 2 diabetes mellitus: systematic review and meta-analysis of randomized and non-randomized studies. BMJ. 2014;348:g2366.
39. US National Library of Medicine. Drug label information: NESINA – alogliptin tablet, film coated. https://dailymed.nlm.nih.gov/dailymed/drugInfo.cfm?setid=a3768c7e-aa4c-44d3-bc53-43bb7346c0b0. Accessed August 8, 2016.
40. Larsson SC, Orsini N, Wolk A. Diabetes mellitus and risk of colorectal cancer: a meta-analysis. J Natl Cancer Inst. 2005;97:1679–87.
41. Huxley R, Ansary-Moghaddam A, de Berrington González A, Barzi F, Woodward M. Type-II diabetes and pancreatic cancer: a meta-analysis of 36 studies. Br J Cancer. 2005;92:2076–83.
42. El-Seraq HB, Hampel H, Javadi F. The association between diabetes and hepatocellular carcinoma: a systematic review of epi-

demiologic   evidence.   Clin   Gastroenterol   Hepatol. 2006;4:369–80.

43. Campbell PT, Newton CC, Patel AV, Jacobs EJ, Gapstur SM. Diabetes and cause-specific mortality in a prospective cohort of one million U.S. adults. Diabetes Care. 2012;35:1835–44.

44. Suissa S, Azoulay L. Metformin and cancer: mounting evidence against an association. Diabetes Care. 2014;37:1786–8.

45. Roberts DL, Dive C, Renehan AG. Biological mechanisms linking obesity and cancer risk: new perspectives. Annu Rev Med. 2010;61:301–16.

46. De Meyts P, Christoffersen CT, Urso B, Wallach B, Grønskov K, Yakushiji F, et al. Role of the time factor in signaling specificity: application to mitogenic and metabolic signaling by the insulin and insulin-like growth factor-I receptor tyrosine kinases. Metabolism. 1995;44:2–11.

47. Vigneri P, Frasca F, Sciacca L, Pandini G, Vigneri R. Diabetes and cancer. Endocr Relat Cancer. 2009;16:1103–23.

48. Vander Heiden MG, Cantley LC, Thompson CB. Understanding the Warburg effect: the metabolic requirements of cell proliferation. Science. 2009;324:1029–33.

49. Handelsman Y, Leroith D, Bloomgarden ZT, Dagogo-Jack S, Einhorn D, Garber AJ, et al. Diabetes and cancer – an AACE/ACE consensus statement. Endocr Pract. 2013;19:675–93.

Chapter 2
Esophageal Disease in Diabetes Mellitus

J. Andy Tau and Lubin Fernando Arevalo Santana

2.1 Esophageal Motility and Diabetes Mellitus

Diabetes mellitus (DM) has multiple clinically important effects on the esophagus. Diabetes results in several esophageal motility disturbances, increases the risk of esophageal candidiasis, and increases the risk of Barrett's esophagus and esophageal carcinoma. Finally, "black esophagus," or acute esophageal necrosis, is also associated with DM. These four entities and their relationship with DM will be reviewed in this section.

Esophageal dysmotility has been shown to be associated with diabetic neuropathy; however, symptomatic esophageal dysmotility is not often considered an important complication of diabetes. Plainly, dysphagia ascribed to diabetic neuropathy should be a diagnosis of exclusion. The effects of blood glucose levels on esophageal motility can be reliably predicted. When blood glucose is increased to 145 mg/dL (physiologic postprandial levels in seen nondiabetic patients),

J.A. Tau (✉) • L.F. Arevalo Santana, MD
Baylor College of Medicine, Department of Medicine, Section of Gastroenterology and Hepatology, Houston, TX, USA
e-mail: tau@bcm.edu; lubin.arevalosantana@bcm.edu

J. Sellin (ed.), *Managing Gastrointestinal Complications of Diabetes*, DOI 10.1007/978-3-319-48662-8_2,
© Springer International Publishing AG 2017

peristalsis velocity increases. However, when increased to 270 mg/dL (pathologic level as seen in patients with diabetes), peristalsis slows and lower esophageal sphincter pressures decrease [1, 2].

In general, the manometric effects of diabetes on the esophagus are not specific and mostly related to speed and strength of peristalsis. While various studies have found differing results, the most consistent changes have been the following:

- Lower pressures/amplitude of esophageal body [3].
- Lower esophagus resting pressure was reduced in patients with longer diabetes duration [4].
- Reduced velocity of esophageal contractions. In other words, the time required for a peristalsis to traverse the esophagus is prolonged [5].
- Frequent spontaneous or multiple peaked body contractions [6].
- Incomplete emptying of the esophagus has been demonstrated in barium and radioisotope studies [7, 8].

Again these findings are nonspecific and can be found in variety of other conditions, such as scleroderma, gastroesophageal reflux disease (GERD), alcoholic neuropathy, and intestinal pseudo-obstruction or ileus. Therefore, other causes should be excluded before ascribing esophageal symptoms (dysphagia, chest pain) to diabetic neuropathy. These changes in motility are likely happening silently. In diabetes, the neuropathologic changes in the esophagus include:

- Segmental demyelination (Schwann cell loss) and axonal degeneration of preganglionic parasympathetic fibers of the vagus nerve [8]. This includes both a reduction in motor vagal ganglions and sensory sympathetic ganglions [9].
- Preservation of the myenteric plexus. This differentiates the pathophysiology from that of achalasia and Chagas disease and explains why diabetic neuropathy alone is rarely the cause of dysphagia.

The pathological findings which amount to loss of cholinergic stimulation are consistent with the manometric findings in the esophagus, which are primarily related to slowed or weakened peristalsis. With preservation of the myenteric plexus, the major regulator of motility in the esophagus, dysphagia is rare. These discoveries were made in historical studies using bethanechol, a cholinergic agent that reliably stimulates the smooth muscle of the esophagus. In achalasia and Chagas disease, bethanechol induced a hypersensitive reaction of the smooth muscles of the esophagus [10], while in diabetics, the hypersensitivity to this drug was not seen [3].

In addition to the autonomic nervous system, via studies mostly in animal models, it is becoming apparent that several parts of enteric nervous system including enteric neurons, interstitial cells of Cajal, glial cells, smooth muscle cells, neurotransmitters, and growth factors are affected by diabetes. Multiple proposed complex mechanisms including oxidative stress, alteration in growth factors, apoptosis, and dysregulation of microRNAs and microbiota have been described [11]. While these discoveries are fledgling, they suggest that therapeutic approaches may need to cover more than one pathophysiologic process to be successful. While there is no therapy beyond the treatment of underlying diabetes, it cannot be overstated that if one is searching for an explanation for dysphagia in a patient with diabetes, diabetes itself is rarely the lone explanation.

2.2   GERD and Diabetes Mellitus

The association between DM and GERD is complex and conflicting. A number of studies have indicated a positive association between GERD and DM, while others have found none. A recent meta-analysis suggests an overall positive association in Western countries [12].

Obesity and concomitant gastroparesis are obvious confounders in this association. Obesity increases intragastric pressure, gastroesophageal gradient, transient lower esophageal sphincter relaxation (TLESR), and esophageal acid exposure, while gastroparesis also increases post-ingestion transient relaxations of the lower esophageal sphincter (LES), producing a greater number of gastroesophageal reflux episodes. The underlying pathogenesis of DM contributing to GERD is not fully elucidated, but is likely related to reduced acid clearance due to slow, weakened esophageal peristalsis.

The association between DM and gastroesophageal reflux (GER) is well established, but the link between DM and GERD, which requires symptoms or esophagitis, is more complex because sensation may be blunted in diabetics with neuropathy. Asymptomatic gastroesophageal reflux (GER) confirmed by pH studies is significantly more frequent in diabetic patients than in healthy controls [13]. In a cohort of patients with varying duration of diabetes, GER (24 h pH monitoring) and esophageal motility (manometry) disorders worsened with long duration of diabetes [14]. Likewise, high-resolution esophageal manometry studies demonstrated lower esophageal resting pressures in patients with longer duration of diabetes [4].

However, whether these pH and manometry findings translate to clinical symptoms or esophagitis (i.e., GERD) is less obvious. Studies have shown that diabetic patients with neuropathy report significantly more GERD symptoms than those without neuropathy [15–17], yet other studies report that GERD symptoms among patients with diabetes are poorly related to neuropathic complications [18, 19]. One possible explanation for this discordance in symptoms and DM is the presence of concomitant sensory neuropathy. For example, two studies have demonstrated that diabetics with neuropathy have evidence of sensory dysfunction based on delayed or extinguished cortical evoked potentials [20, 21]. These studies indicate that diabetics with afferent nerve damage have increased sensory thresholds for pain or symptoms in the esophagus. Thus, while they may have more acid exposure and less acid clearance, sensory neuropathy may blunt the symptoms. Thus, long-standing diabetics with neuropathy are at higher risk for GERD even if they have no symptoms.

2.3 Barrett's Esophagus, Esophageal Cancer, and Diabetes Mellitus

Diabetes mellitus may be a risk factor for Barrett's esophagus (BE) and esophageal cancer independent of GERD and obesity. In a population-based retrospective case-control study using the General Practice Research Database, a UK primary care database that contains information on more than eight million subjects, type 2 DM was found to be a risk factor for BE, independent of obesity, smoking, or a diagnosis of GERD [22]. On multivariable analysis, diabetes was associated with a 49 % increase in the risk of BE, independent of other known risk factors (odds ratio, 1.49; 95 % confidence interval [CI], 1.16–1.91). In a meta-analysis, including six case-control studies and 11 cohort studies, individuals with DM had a modestly increased risk of EC, in particular adenocarcinoma (summary relative risk [SRR] 2.12, 95 % CI, 1.01–4.46) [23]. These studies suggest that independent of the mechanical effects of obesity and GERD, metabolic pathways related to diabetes itself play a role in the pathogenesis of Barrett's and esophageal carcinogenesis. For example, one theory postulates that elevated insulin concentrations in diabetics lower concentrations of IGF-binding proteins (IGFBPs), which in turn contribute to an upregulated level of insulin-like growth factors (IGFs), which stimulate growth through cellular proliferation and inhibition of apoptosis within the esophageal carcinoma cells [24]. In vitro studies, animal models, and epidemiologic data have demonstrated the role of insulin-like growth factor 1 (IGF-1) in carcinogenesis of the esophagus [25]. The risk appears to be most highly associated with adenocarcinoma, as a recent study failed to demonstrate an association of squamous cell carcinoma and diabetes [26].

Esophageal Candidiasis and Diabetes Mellitus

Diabetes is considered as a risk factor for esophageal candidiasis (EC) because of impaired immunity and stasis of esophageal contents. Most cases are associated with chronically poor glycemic control. Esophageal colonization with candida is commonplace as it is a normal mouth flora, occurring up to 20 % of normal healthy patients. However, esophagitis requires deeper invasion of the mucosa. It has been demonstrated in multiple case reports that underlying diabetes was the only predisposing factor for the development of candida esophagitis [27]. The pathogenesis is believed to be a combination of:

- Prolonged emptying of the esophagus, allowing for increased colonization.
- Defective cellular immunity (specifically, impaired chemotaxis and phagocytosis) [28, 29].
- Increased fungal virulence in high glucose environments in diabetics. Specifically, *Candida albicans* expresses a surface protein that has significant homology with the receptor for complement factor 3b, which has increased expression in hyperglycemic settings, resulting in competitive binding and inhibition of the complement-mediated phagocytosis [30].
- Increased adherence to diabetic cells due to alteration in the carbohydrate composition of receptors of the epithelium. This has been demonstrated in the buccal mucosa (thrush) in DM and presumed to occur in the esophageal mucosa [31].

The clinical presentation varies from scattered white plaques without symptoms to dense pseudomembranous plaques and erosions with severe odynophagia or dysphagia. The preferred treatment is fluconazole 200–400 mg PO/IV daily for 14–21 days. More severe disease can be treated with an echinocandin or amphotericin B deoxycholate 0.3–0.7 mg/kg. Other oral alternatives include itraconazole 200 mg daily, posaconazole 400 mg b.i.d, or voriconazole 200 mg b.i.d.

2.4   Black Esophagus and Diabetes Mellitus

Black esophagus, or acute esophageal necrosis, is a rare syndrome that arises from ischemic insult from hypotension, corrosive injury from gastric acid, and decreased function of mucosal barrier in malnourished and debilitated patients. It is most commonly seen in critically ill patients with sepsis, diabetic ketoacidosis, multi-organ failure, massive thromboembolic disease, severe trauma, or malignancy. Diabetes appears to be a risk factor with approximately 24–28 % of patients who develop "black esophagus" having underlying DM [32, 33]. Patients typically present with upper gastrointestinal hemorrhage. Diffuse circumferential black mucosal discoloration in the distal esophagus arising from the GE junction is the hallmark appearance of "black esophagus." The treatment is directed at the underlying cause of the critical illness and control of hyperglycemia. Antacids and parenteral nutrition have been used as supportive measures, but have not been studied singularly [34].

2.5   Conclusion

Diabetes-related esophageal dysmotility does not cause dysphagia, but DM appears to be a risk factor for GERD, Barrett's esophagus, and esophageal carcinoma. Abnormal pH and motility studies do not correlate very well with the GI symptoms of diabetics, possibly due to DM-related sensory dysfunction. Poorly controlled DM is associated with both the white plaques of esophageal candidiasis and the black esophagus of acute esophageal necrosis occasionally seen in the critically ill.

References

1. De Boer SY, Masclee AAM, Lam WF, Lamers CBHW. Effect of acute hyperglycemia on esophageal motility and lower esophageal sphincter pressure in humans. Gastroenterology. 1992;103:775–80.
2. Boeckxstaens GE, Horowitz M, Bermingham H, Holloway RH. Physiological variations in blood glucose concentration affect oesophageal motility and sensation in normal subjects. Neurogastroenterol Motil. 1997;9:239–46.

3. Stewart IM, Hosking DJ, Preston BJ, Atkinson M. Oesophageal motor changes in diabetes mellitus. Thorax. 1976;31:278–83.
4. Boronikolos GC, Menge BA, Schenker N, Breuer TGK, Otte J-M, et al. Upper gastrointestinal motility and symptoms in individuals with diabetes, prediabetes and normal glucose tolerance. Diabetologia. 2015;58:1175–82.
5. Hollis JB, Castell DO, Braddom RL. Esophageal motor function in diabetes mellitus and its relationship to peripheral neuropathy. Gastroenterology. 1977;73:1098–102.
6. Loo FD, Dodds WJ, Soergel KH, Arndorfer RC, Helm JF, Hogan WJ. Multipeaked esophageal peristaltic pressure waves in patients with diabetic neuropathy. Gastroenterology. 1985;88:485–91.
7. Russell CO, Gannan R, Coatsworth J, Neilsen R, Allen F, Hill LD, Pope CEI. Relationship among esophageal dysfunction, diabetic gastroenteropathy and peripheral neuropathy. Dig Dis Sci. 1983;28:289–93.
8. Guy RJ, Dawson JL, Garrett JR, Laws JW, Thomas PK, Sharma AK, Watkins PJ. Diabetic gastroparesis from autonomic neuropathy: surgical considerations and changes in vagus nerve morphology. J Neurol Neurosurg Psychiatry. 1984;47:686–91.
9. Carroll SL, Byer SJ, Dorsey DA, Watson MA, Schmidt RE. Ganglion-specific patterns of diabetes modulated gene expression are established in prevertebral and paravertebral sympathetic ganglia prior to the development of neuroaxonal dystrophy. J Neuropathol Exp Neurol. 2004;63:1144–54.
10. Heitmann P, Espinoza J. Oesophageal manometric studies in patients with chronic Chagas disease and megacolon. Gut. 1969;10:848–51.
11. Yarandi SS, Srinivasan S. Diabetic gastrointestinal motility disorders and the role of enteric nervous system: current status and future directions. Neurogastroenterol Motil. 2014;26:611–24.
12. Sun X-M, Tan J-C, Zhu Y, Lin L. Association between diabetes mellitus and gastroesophageal reflux disease: a meta-analysis. WJG. 2015;21:3085–92.
13. Lluch I, Ascaso JF, Mora F, Minguez M, Pena A, Hernandez A, et al. Gastroesophageal reflux in diabetes mellitus. Am J Gastroenterol. 1999;94:919–24.
14. Kinekawa F, Kubo F, Matsuda K, Fujita Y, Tomita T, Uchida Y, Nishioka M. Relationship between esophageal dysfunction and neuropathy in diabetic patients. Am J Gastroenterol. 2001;96:2026–32.

15. Wang X, Pitchumoni CS, Chandrarana K, Shah N. Increased prevalence of symptoms of gastroesophageal reflux diseases in type 2 diabetics with neuropathy. World J Gastroenterol. 2008;14:709–12.
16. Nishida T, Tsuji S, Tsujii M, Arimitsu S, Sato T, Haruna Y, et al. Gastroesophageal reflux disease related to diabetes: analysis of 241 cases with type 2 diabetes mellitus. J Gastroenterol Hepatol. 2004;19:258–65.
17. Spångéus A, El-Salhy M, Suhr O, Eriksson J, Lithner F. Prevalence of gastrointestinal symptoms in young and middle-aged diabetic patients. Scand J Gastroenterol. 1999;34:1196–202.
18. Clouse RE, Lustman PJ. Gastrointestinal symptoms in diabetic patients: lack of association with neuropathy. Am J Gastroenterol. 1989;84:868–72.
19. Lee SD, Keum B, Chun HJ, Bak YT. Gastroesophageal reflux disease in type II diabetes mellitus with or without peripheral neuropathy. J Neurogastroenterol Motil. 2011;17:274–8.
20. Rathmann W, Enck P, Frieling T, Gries FA. Visceral afferent neuropathy in diabetic gastroparesis. Diabetes Care. 1991;14:1086–9.
21. Kamath MV, Tougas G, Fitzpatrick D, Fallen EL, Watteel R, Shine G, et al. Assessment of the visceral afferent and autonomic pathways in response to esophageal stimulation in control subjects and in patients with diabetes. Clin Invest Med. 1998;21:100–13.
22. Iyer PG, Borah BJ, Heien HC, et al. Association of Barrett's esophagus with type II Diabetes Mellitus: results from a large population-based case-control study. Clinical Gastroenterology &Hepatology. 2013;11:1108–1114.
23. Huang W, Ren H, Ben Q, Cai Q, Zhu W, Li Z. Risk of esophageal cancer in diabetes mellitus: a meta-analysis of observational studies. Cancer Causes Control. 2012;23:263–72.
24. Juan HC, Tsai HT, Chang PH, Huang CY, Hu CP, Wong FH. Insulin-like growth factor 1 mediates 5-fluorouracil chemoresistance in esophageal carcinoma cells through increasing survivin stability. Apoptosis. 2011;16:174–83.
25. McElholm AR, McKnight AJ, Patterson CC, Johnston BT, Hardie LJ, Murray LJ. A population-based study of IGF axis polymorphisms and the esophageal inflammation, metaplasia, adenocarcinoma sequence. Gastroenterology. 2010;139:204–12.
26. Cheng KC, Chen YL, Lai SW, Tsai PY, Sung FC. Risk of esophagus cancer in diabetes mellitus: a population-based case-control study in Taiwan. BMC Gastroenterol. 2012;12:177.

27. Takasawa H, Takahashi Y, Abe M, Osame K, Watanabe S, Hisatake T, et al. An elderly case of type 2 diabetes which developed in association with oral and esophageal candidiasis. Intern Med. 2007;46:387–90.
28. Hostetter MK. Perspectives in diabetes. Handicaps to host defense. Effects of hyperglycemia on C3 and *Candida albicans*. Diabetes. 1990;39:271–5.
29. Tan JS, Anderson JL, Watanakunakorn C, Phair JP. Neutrophil dysfunction in diabetes mellitus. J Lab Clin Med. 1975;85:26–33.
30. Deresinski S. Infections in the diabetic patient: strategies for the clinician. Infect Dis Rep. 1995;1:1–12.
31. Darwazeh AMG, Lamey PJ, Samaranayake LP, MacFarlane TW, Fisher BM, MacRury SM, Maccuish AC. The relationship between colonisation, secretor status and in vitro adhesion of *Candida albicans* to buccal epithelial cells from diabetics. J Med Microbiol. 1990;33:43–9.
32. Gurvits GE, Shapsis A, Lau N, Gualtieri N, Robilotti JG. Acute esophageal necrosis: a rare syndrome. J Gastroenterol. 2007;42:29–38.
33. Grudell AB, Mueller PS, Viggiano TR. Black esophagus: report of six cases and review of the literature, 1963–2003. Dis Esophagus. 2006;19:105–10.
34. Carneiro M, Lescano M, Romanello L. Acute esophageal necrosis. Dig Endosc. 2005;17:89–92.

Chapter 3
Diabetic Gastroparesis

Aylin Tansel and Nisreen Husain

3.1 Introduction

Gastroparesis is defined as a chronic disorder characterized by delayed emptying of the stomach occurring in the absence of mechanical obstruction. It is a well-known and potentially serious complication of diabetes. Although gastroparesis was initially described in patients with type 1 diabetes, it is increasingly being recognized in patients with type 2 diabetes. Diabetic gastroparesis affects up to 40 % of patients with type 1 diabetes and up to 30 % of patients with type 2 diabetes [1, 2]. Diabetic gastroparesis generally affects patients with long-standing diabetes mellitus, and patients often have other diabetic complications such as retinopathy, neuropathy, or nephropathy. Gastroparesis can lead to poor glucose control, increased morbidity, and decreased quality of life. As the number of patients with diabetes increases, the number of diabetic patients with gastroparesis is increasing. For reasons that remain unclear, approximately 80 % of patients with gastroparesis are women [3]. Hospitalizations with gastroparesis as the primary diagnosis have increased 158 % from 1995 to 2004 [4].

A. Tansel • N. Husain
Section of Gastroenterology and Hepatology, Department of Medicine, Baylor College of Medicine and Michael E. DeBakey Veterans Affairs Medical Center, Houston, TX, USA
e-mail: nisreenh@bcm.edu

J. Sellin (ed.), *Managing Gastrointestinal Complications of Diabetes*, DOI 10.1007/978-3-319-48662-8_3,
© Springer International Publishing AG 2017

Additionally, gastroparesis has the longest length of stay when compared with other upper gastrointestinal conditions [4]. This chapter will explore the clinical features, complications, diagnosis, management, and treatment options for gastroparesis.

3.2   Clinical Features

In diabetes, delayed gastric emptying can often be asymptomatic. Therefore, the term gastroparesis should only be reserved for patients that have both delayed gastric emptying and upper gastrointestinal symptoms. Additionally, discordance between the pattern and type of symptoms and the magnitude of delayed gastric emptying is a well-established phenomenon. Accelerating gastric emptying may not improve symptoms, and patients can have symptomatic improvement while gastric emptying time remains unchanged. Furthermore, patients with severe symptoms can have mild delays in gastric emptying.

Clinical features of gastroparesis include nausea, vomiting, bloating, abdominal pain, and malnutrition. In a tertiary care center of 146 patients, nausea was present in 92 %, vomiting in 84 %, abdominal bloating in 75 %, and early satiety in 60 % of patients [3]. Functional dyspepsia and gastroparesis have significant overlap, and up to 50 % of patients with dyspeptic symptoms can have delayed gastric emptying [5]. Abdominal pain is present in 46–89 % of patients and is often difficult to treat [3]. Impaired regulation of postprandial glycemia can also be an indication of gastroparesis. Gastroparesis affects oral drug absorption and can cause hyperglycemia that is challenging to manage, in addition to unexplained hypoglycemia. As a result, unstable glucose control can be a subtle sign of gastroparesis.

3.3   Complications

Gastroparesis can lead to poor nutrition and poor oral intake with subsequent malnutrition and vitamin and mineral deficiencies. Possible complications of gastroparesis include volume depletion with renal failure, malnutrition, electrolyte abnormalities, esophagitis, Mallory–Weiss tear (from vomiting), or bezoar formation. Patients with gastroparesis will often have other gastrointestinal manifestations of delayed motility.

3.3.1   Nutrition

Nutritional and caloric deficits are common in patients with gastroparesis, and patients should receive nutritional screening. In a study of 305 patients, 64 % of patients were found to have caloric deficient diets, defined as less than 60 % of daily total energy requirements [6]. One study of 45 patients found that foods provoking symptoms were generally fatty, acidic, spicy, and roughage based [7]. Additionally, patients were found to have several vitamin and mineral deficiencies specifically vitamins A, B6, C, and K, iron, potassium, and zinc [6]. Nutritional consultation increases the chances that daily total energy requirements will be met (odds ratio = 1.51, $P = 0.08$) [6]. Unfortunately, despite known nutritional and caloric deficiencies, nutritional consultation is often neglected, and only a minority receives a nutritional consultation [6].

3.3.2   Glycemic Control and Gastroparesis

It has been well documented that acute changes in blood glucose alter gastric emptying [8]. Additionally, acute hyperglycemia can attenuate the effect of prokinetics reducing their efficacy. Induction of acute hypoglycemia accelerates gastric emptying. Glucose control is often complicated in patients with diabetic gastroparesis as blood glucose levels both influence and are influenced by gastroparesis [9]. Long-term hyperglycemia is an independent risk factor for gastroparesis [8]. However, it has been shown that long-term glycemic control does not improve gastric emptying [8, 10].

3.4   Diagnosis

A diagnosis of gastroparesis should only be made in patients that have both upper gastrointestinal symptoms and objective evidence of delayed gastric emptying. Diabetic gastroparesis is diagnosed by demonstrating delayed gastric emptying in a symptomatic patient after the exclusion of other etiologies of symptoms and exclusion of mechanical obstruction. An upper endoscopy is important to exclude the presence of ulcer, stricture, or mass.

Initial investigation should include a complete blood count, complete metabolic profile, and thyroid-stimulating hormone. Additionally, a pregnancy test should be obtained in women of childbearing age. If vomiting or pain is acute or severe, consider an abdominal obstruction series. If abdominal pain is a significant symptom, workup may include a right upper quadrant ultrasound, amylase, and lipase. Once mechanical obstruction has been excluded, gastroparesis is diagnosed by demonstrating delayed gastric emptying with solid phase gastric emptying scintigraphy, wireless motility capsule (SmartPill), or stable isotope breath test.

3.4.1   Gastric Emptying Scintigraphy

The gold standard to evaluate delayed gastric emptying is a solid phase gastric emptying scintigraphy over 4 h. The Society of Nuclear Medicine and American Neurogastroenterology and Motility Society (ANMS) has a standardized protocol for gastric emptying scintigraphy [11]. It is important that it is performed with a solid meal because liquid emptying may remain normal despite advanced disease. The standardized meal for testing is 99-m technetium sulfur-colloid labeled low fat, egg white. The scan should be performed with the patient in an upright position 1, 2, and 4 h after the test meal to identify both rapid and slow gastric emptying. Prior to testing, medications that can impair or promote gastric emptying should be held at least 48–72 h in advance. Patients already taking prokinetics should stop taking them prior to testing. Medications that delay gastric emptying and should be held include narcotic analgesics, tricyclic antidepressants, lithium, and calcium channel blockers. Serotonin receptor antagonists, such as ondansetron, can be given during testing for severe symptoms of nausea and vomiting because they do not alter gastric emptying. Table 3.1 provides a more complete list of medications that affect gastric emptying.

Interpreting the results of a gastric emptying study can be challenging in patients with diabetes. Hyperglycemia has been shown to result in delayed gastric emptying on scintigraphy, and gastric emptying normalized when euglycemia was achieved prior to testing [12]. It may be advisable to check glucose levels prior to a gastric emptying study to ensure that glucose levels are within normal range [13]. Ideally blood glucose levels in patients with diabetes should be <275 mg/dL on the day of the test because hyperglycemia significantly delays gastric emptying [13, 14].

One disadvantage of gastric emptying scintigraphy is that it is often not performed in a standardized manner in many

TABLE 3.1 Medications that affect gastric emptying

Delay gastric emptying	Accelerate gastric emptying
Opiates (e.g., oxycodone, acetaminophen–codeine)	Macrolide antibiotics (e.g., erythromycin, azithromycin, clarithromycin)
Anticholinergics (e.g., dicyclomine, hyoscyamine, tricyclic antidepressants such as amitriptyline)	Metoclopramide
Aluminum-containing antacids	Diazepam
Dopamine, levodopa	Bulk laxatives
Calcium channel blockers (e.g., diltiazem, verapamil, nifedipine)	
GLP analogue (e.g., exenatide)	

medical centers. Despite strong guidelines that scintigraphy be performed over 4 h, many medical centers continue to extrapolate gastric emptying using data after 90–120 min. Results from scintigraphy tests under 4 h long should not be used to diagnose gastroparesis. Another disadvantage of this test is radiation exposure. The amount of exposure with testing is equivalent to approximately one-third of the average annual radiation exposure in the United States from natural sources [13].

3.4.2   Wireless Motility Capsule

The SmartPill® GI Monitoring System (SmartPill Corporation, NY, USA) is an ingested capsule that can also be used to diagnose gastroparesis. The pill is swallowed after ingesting a standardized meal and delivers information on pressure, pH, and temperature wirelessly to a data recorder worn by the patient. The data estimates gastric emptying time, combined small and large bowel transit time, and total transit time and studies pressure patterns in the stomach, small bowel, and colon. The capsule is approved by the US Food and Drug Administration for use in studying gastroparesis. In a study of 87 healthy controls and 61 patients with gastroparesis, the wireless motility capsule had a sensitivity of 87 % and specificity of 92 % when compared with a 4-h scintigraphic gastric emptying test [15]. The device is a reasonable alternative to conventional scintigraphy for gastroparesis but is not widely available. Advantages of this test are the ambulatory measure of the test, lack of radiation exposure, and ability to measure motility of the entire GI tract. Disadvantages of this test are the cost and lack of availability.

3.4.3 CO_2 Breath Test

Another diagnostic option is the stable isotope breath test. 13C-labeled octanoate, a medium-chain triglyceride, is bound to a solid meal. After ingestion, 13C-labeled octanoate is quickly absorbed in the small intestine and metabolized to 13CO2 which is excreted from the lungs. This test is less expensive than scintigraphy and avoids radiation exposure which can be beneficial to certain populations (i.e., pregnancy, breastfeeding, children). Disadvantages of this test are the need for normal small intestinal absorption, normal liver metabolism, and the need to assess pulmonary excretion to detect radioactivity. Furthermore, this test is currently not available for clinical use in the United States.

3.5   Initial Treatment

Treatment should be tailored for each patient based on symptoms. Disease severity is assessed by the patients' ability to maintain adequate nutrition and by symptoms. A daily diary of symptoms and diet may be helpful to assess severity of symptoms of gastroparesis for patients with difficulty remembering symptoms. The Gastroparesis Cardinal Symptom Index (GCSI), a validated scoring system shown in Table 3.2,

TABLE 3.2 Gastroparesis Cardinal Symptom Index (GCSI)

	None	Very mild	Mild	Moderate	Severe	Very severe
Nausea	0	1	2	3	4	5
Retching	0	1	2	3	4	5
Vomiting	0	1	2	3	4	5
Stomach fullness	0	1	2	3	4	5
Not able to finish a normal-sized meal	0	1	2	3	4	5
Feel excessively full after meals	0	1	2	3	4	5
Loss of appetite	0	1	2	3	4	5
Bloating	0	1	2	3	4	5
Belly visible larger	0	1	2	3	4	5

can assess the severity of gastroparesis as well as response to management [16]. Figure 3.1 provides a pyramid of treatment, with progression up the pyramid as severity of gastroparesis increases [17]. Patients with mild gastroparesis can be managed with dietary modifications, glucose control, and symptom management.

Elevated glucose levels have a significant role in slowing gastric emptying. Changes in gastric emptying may affect postprandial blood glucose concentrations, because of unpredictable delivery of food. Impaired gastric emptying with continued administration of exogenous insulin

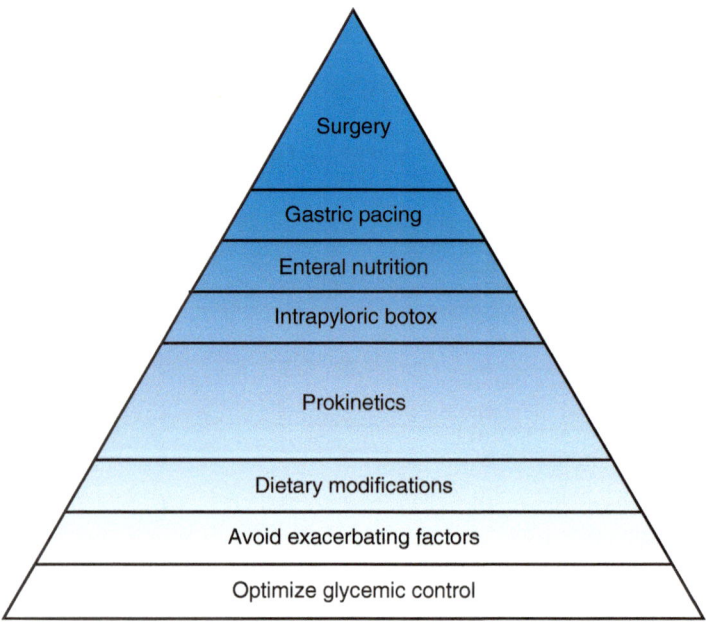

FIGURE 3.1 Therapeutic pyramid for diabetic gastroparesis. Starting at the base, patients with mild symptoms can be managed with glycemic control and dietary modifications. The peak of the pyramid represents the minority of patients that do not respond to therapy, and therapeutic options are limited and not necessarily evidence based (Reproduced with permission from Sellin [17] ©Nature)

can cause hypoglycemia. Therefore, in patients with established gastroparesis, short-acting insulin should be dosed *after* rather than *prior* to meals to avoid hypoglycemia. The use of regular insulin rather than rapid-acting insulin analogues may be better as it has a sustained duration of action.

3.5.1 Dietary Treatment

Initial treatment should be dietary management with a low-fat, low-fiber diet with small frequent meals. By eating meals more frequently, patients are more likely to continue to meet their nutrition needs. Large meals lead to longer gastric emptying, so by decreasing the volume of meals, patients may experience some relief in symptoms. Fat is known to slow gastric emptying and fiber can increase risk for bezoar formation. Food should be chewed thoroughly and meal replacement drinks should be considered. Patients should sit up while eating and for 1 h after finishing their meal. Multivitamin supplementation is advisable. Foods that are acidic, spicy, high in fat, and roughage based can increase overall symptoms in patients with gastroparesis. Patients should avoid alcohol and smoking as these can delay gastric emptying [18, 19]. Table 3.3 provides suggested nutrition guidelines.

If solid food is not tolerated, patients can try blended foods. In many cases, normal gastric emptying of liquids is preserved despite delayed gastric emptying of solids. Prior to blending, solid foods should be thinned with some type of liquid such as water, low-fat milk, or broth. If patients are not consuming enough calories, then patients should supplement their diet with nutritional supplements. Indications for nutritional supplementation include weight loss of greater than or equal to 10 % during a period of 3–6 months, inability to maintain recommended body weight, and severe symptoms requiring hospitalization or interventions such as a nasogastric tube to relieve nausea and vomiting [20].

TABLE 3.3 Nutritional interventions

1. Decrease volume of meals

2. Improve glycemic control

3. Limit fat

(a) Fat in liquid form is well tolerated; maintain 20–30 % of calories from fat

4. Limit fiber

(a) Identify high-fiber foods that increase upper gastrointestinal symptoms

(b) If bezoar formation is a concern, avoid foods causing bezoar such as oranges, berries, coconut, and legumes

(c) Fiber supplements for constipation should be discontinued

5. Meal consistency

(a) Chew food thoroughly and take 20–30 min to finish meal

(b) If solids are not tolerated, any food can be blended with water, low-fat milk, vegetable juice, or broth to make a puree

(i) Liquid nutrients are better tolerated than solid food

(ii) Can also try solid foods in the morning, switch to semiliquid and/or liquid meals over the course of the day

6. Additional recommendations

(a) Monitor and replace micronutrients as needed: iron, vitamin B12, vitamin D, calcium

(b) Avoid caffeine, alcohol, and tobacco

(c) Eat nutritious foods prior to filling-up on "empty calories"

(d) Avoid foods that lower esophageal sphincter pressure: peppermint, chocolate, fat, caffeine

(e) Chew well and eat slowly (30-min meals)

(f) Do not lie down immediately after eating – sit upright or consider walking for 1–2 h after meals

(g) If overweight, lose weight

(h) On days when symptoms are worse, just take liquids to let the stomach rest

(i) Check weight twice a week; if weight is decreasing, increase the amount of liquid supplements

3.6   Pharmacologic Treatments

When dietary management and glycemic control are not sufficient to control symptoms, pharmacologic treatment should be initiated. Initial pharmacologic treatment should be with prokinetic agent and/or antiemetic agent. If there is no clinical response to these medications, then consider further investigation by a gastroenterologist. Unfortunately, there is a dearth of medications available to treat gastroparesis. Additionally, many of the medications used are based on older trials with small sample sizes. Table 3.4 provides a short summary of medications.

3.6.1   Prokinetics

Pharmacological therapy is necessary in patients that have continued symptoms despite dietary modification. The mainstay of pharmacological therapy is prokinetic agents.

The only Food and Drug Administration (FDA)-approved medication for gastroparesis in the United States is metoclopramide, which has both prokinetic and antiemetic effects. Metoclopramide, a central and peripheral dopamine 2 (D2) receptor antagonist and 5-hydroxytryptamine (5-HT) receptor agonist, works by increasing antral contractions, decreasing fundal relaxation, and improving antroduodenal coordination. Metoclopramide was established as effective based on four placebo-controlled trials that improved gastric emptying and symptoms [21–24].

These studies were not conducted for longer than 4 weeks. Up to 30 % of patients taking metoclopramide experience side effects. Metoclopramide crosses the blood–brain barrier and is therefore associated with neurological symptoms in up to 10 % of patients. The most common neurologic side effect is a Parkinson's-type syndrome which is reversible 2–3 months after discontinuation of the drug. However, one particularly concerning side effect is tardive dyskinesia. Tardive dyskinesia is irreversible and occurs in 1 % of cases when metoclopramide is taken for more than 3 months [25]. Since

TABLE 3.4 Medications to treat diabetic gastroparesis

Drug class	Medication	Route	Dosing	Side effects
D2 receptor antagonist, 5-HT3 receptor antagonist, 5-HT4 receptor agonist	Metoclopramide	PO, IV, SC, IM	5–20 mg TID or QID before meals (and at bedtime)	Anxiety, depression, galactorrhea, extrapyramidal movement disorders, tardive dyskinesia
D2/D3 receptor antagonist (peripheral)	Domperidone	PO	10–20 mg TID before meals and at bedtime	Hyperprolactinemia, breast tenderness, galactorrhea
Motilin receptor agonist[a]	Erythromycin	PO, IV, IV formulation more effective than PO	125–250 mg PO BID or TID before meals 3 mg/kg IV q8 hr	Abdominal cramping, early satiety, rashes, urticaria, nausea, diarrhea
5-HT3 receptor antagonist	Ondansetron	PO, IV	4–8 mg BID or TID	Headache, increased liver enzymes, constipation
Phenothiazine	Prochlorperazine	PO, PR	5–10 mg PO TID 5–25 mg PR q12 hr	Hypotension, extrapyramidal symptoms

[a]Contraindicated with P450 3A4 inhibitors (e.g., grapefruit juice, antifungal agents, cisapride, anticancer drugs such as tamoxifen, antidepressants such as fluoxetine and midazolam, agents against the human immunodeficiency virus such as ritonavir, or antihypertensive agents such as verapamil). [28, 53]

2009, there has been an FDA black box warning against use beyond 3 months unless benefit outweighs the risk. If a patient desires to continue longer than 3 months, informed consent should be obtained. Development of tardive dyskinesia is related to the duration of metoclopramide use and the number of doses taken. People most at risk for developing acute dystonic reactions include women, children, and patients receiving high doses of medication. It is important to carefully monitor patients for the earliest signs of tardive dyskinesia, because discontinuing therapy early may help minimize permanent side effects. The Abnormal Involuntary Movement Scale (AIMS) can be used for early detection of tardive dyskinesia. The AIMS is a 12-item scale that is clinician administered and scored to assess severity (http://www. cqaimh.org/pdf/tool_aims.pdf).

A proposed method for prescribing metoclopramide can be to start a test dose (i.e., 5 mg 15 min before meals and at bedtime), titrating to the lowest efficacious dose and instituting dose reductions (i.e., 5 mg before two main meals of the day) or drug holidays whenever possible. An alternative method is to start at 5–10 mg two to three times daily and increase as tolerated up to 10–20 mg three to four times daily. If there is clinical response, maintain lowest effective dose. In patients with persistent symptoms, consider a short course of erythromycin (250–500 mg daily). If there are significant side effects, domperidone 10 mg three times daily (up to 20 mg four times daily) can be used.

Intranasal metoclopramide is a potentially promising treatment with a potentially lower side effect profile. An advantage of the nasal spray is that it is absorbed even when patients have delayed gastric emptying or nausea and vomiting. A recent multicenter double-blind study of metoclopramide nasal spray found significant reduction of symptoms among women, but not men, with diabetic gastroparesis [26].

Domperidone is a peripheral dopamine D2 and D3 receptor antagonist and is equally efficacious as metoclopramide. Unlike metoclopramide, it crosses the blood–brain barrier poorly and, therefore, has fewer CNS side effects than meto-clopramide. As a result, it is emerging as the oral drug of choice, particularly in older patients. It is a good alternative if patients have significant neurologic side effects with metoclo-pramide. Despite evidence that domperidone is equally effi-cacious and safer than metoclopramide, it is not approved by the FDA for prescription in the United States. However, domperidone is available in the United States through the Investigational New Drug Program.

Erythromycin is a motilin receptor agonist and is the most potent drug to accelerate gastric emptying when given intra-venously. Therefore, intravenous erythromycin is often the initial treatment for patients hospitalized with gastroparesis. Orally administered erythromycin tends to be less effective than intravenous administration. Elixir form of erythromycin may have better absorption and bioavailability than pill forms. The treatment effect generally decreases after 4 weeks and chronic use can lead to tachyphylaxis. If tachyphylaxis develops, erythromycin can be discontinued for at least 2 weeks and then restarted. In a large cohort, erythromycin doubled the risk of sudden death from cardiac causes com-pared to a control population [27]. Furthermore, the risk for death was increased in patients on medications that were cytochrome P450 3A inhibitors which include nitroimidazole antifungal agents, diltiazem, verapamil, and troleandomycin [27]. Erythromycin is best used for exacerbations or intermit-tently if patients are unable to tolerate or respond to meto-clopramide or need a drug holiday.

Cisapride and tegaserod are 5-HT receptor 4 agonists that induce the release of acetylcholine from myenteric choliner-gic neurons along the gastrointestinal tract to stimulate gas-tric emptying. Cisapride is more potent than tegaserod. Both medications have been withdrawn from the market because of cardiac complications – mainly cardiac arrhythmias includ-ing torsades de pointes. Cisapride is available through a com-passionate use program through Janssen Pharmaceuticals with strict monitoring guidelines and only when other medi-cations have failed.

3.6.2   Antiemetics

Antiemetics can be used for symptom relief. There are no trials examining effectiveness for gastroparesis. Phenothiazine derivatives (such as promethazine and prochlorperazine) and serotonin antagonists (such as ondansetron and granisetron) can be useful medications for nausea and vomiting symptoms. Other medications that have been used for nausea and vomiting include benzodiazepines (such as lorazepam) and histamine H1 receptor antagonists (such as meclizine, synthetic cannabinoids, and transdermal scopolamine) [28].

3.6.3   Medications for Abdominal Pain

Gastroparesis can be associated with abdominal pain in as many as 50 % of patients with gastroparesis at tertiary care centers. There are no trials to guide the choice of agents. Low-dose tricyclic antidepressants, duloxetine, gabapentin, and pregabalin can be used. A 15-week multicenter parallel group placebo-controlled double-blind randomized clinical trial comparing nortriptyline with placebo for symptomatic relief in idiopathic gastroparesis of 138 patients failed to show significant improvement in symptoms [29]. Tramadol may be considered for refractory symptoms. Opiates should be avoided because of their inhibition on gastric motility and addiction potential.

3.7   Endoscopic and Surgical Management

3.7.1   Botulinum Toxin

Intrapyloric injection of botulinum toxin is thought to decrease pylorospasm associated with gastroparesis and possibly improve symptoms. Several small open-label and retrospective studies showed improvement in symptoms and improvement in gastric emptying [30–34]. However, two small randomized double-blind placebo-controlled trials failed to show benefit between saline injection and botulinum toxin [35, 36]. Because efficacy of botulinum toxin has not been demonstrated effective in prospective double-blind studies, current clinical guidelines do not recommend the use of botulinum toxin. Despite lack of definitive supporting evidence, botulinum toxin is performed at many centers particularly when pyloric dysfunction is suspected. Clinically, there may be some benefit to some patients; however, botulinum toxin injection requires frequent treatments to remain effective.

3.7.2   Gastrostomy/Jejunostomy

Enteral nutrition is recommended in patients with insufficient oral intake, unintentional loss of 10 % or more of body weight during a 3–6-month period, and/or repeated hospitalizations for refractory symptoms [37]. If enteral supplementation may be required for more than 3 months, it is best to provide enteral supplementation through a jejunostomy tube. Enteral nutrition is always preferred to parenteral nutrition, as parenteral nutrition has risks of infection and liver disease. A short-term nasojejunal feeding tube can be used to determine if the patient will tolerate feeding through permanent enteral access. Feeding jejunostomy can be placed to improve symptoms and nutritional status but can be associated with complications such as tube dislocation or migration, bowel obstruction, bleeding, bowel perforation, abdominal wall infection, enterocutaneous fistulas, and intestinal ischemia. Jejunostomy can be placed by open or laparoscopic surgery. It is not advisable to place endoscopically, because of a high rate of tube placement failure and complications [38]. An additional insertion of a venting gastrostomy can additionally improve symptoms of gastroparesis with severe intractable nausea and vomiting.

3.7.3   Gastric Electrical Stimulation

Gastric electrical stimulation (GES) is an increasingly utilized method for treatment. There is one device (Enterra®) that is approved by the FDA with a Humanitarian Device Exemption for patients with refractory symptoms. Gastric electrical stimulation is generally reserved for patients with persistent nausea and vomiting despite medical treatment for at least 1 year. This device produces low-energy high-frequency (12/min) pulses of short duration that do not affect gastric emptying but have been shown to improve symptoms, nutrition, weight, and glycemic control. The mechanism of action is unclear, but the current hypothesis is that GES stimulates afferent pathways to the brain to control nausea and vomiting. The majority of data of the benefits has been from open-label, uncontrolled studies. A prospective study of 151 patients (72 diabetic, 73 idiopathic, 6 others) with refractory gastroparesis found the most clinical improvement in diabetic patients. The symptoms which most significantly improved included nausea, loss of appetite, and early satiety [39]. Following GES placement, patients had significant improvement in total symptom score, nausea severity score, and requirement for enteral or parenteral nutrition [40]. The device removal or reimplantation rate was 8.3 % [40]. This suggests GES is relatively safe and effective; however, controlled studies are required to confirm the clinical benefits.

3.7.4   Surgical Pyloroplasty

There are limited data for pyloroplasty, but small studies suggest surgical pyloroplasty can accelerate gastric emptying and improve symptoms in select patients, particularly those with refractory symptoms and clinical suspicion for pyloric dysfunction. The two largest studies showed clinical improvement of 82 % and 83 %, respectively; however, there are no randomized trials to evaluate pyloroplasty [41, 42].

3.7.5   Gastrectomy

This is reserved as a last resort and there is limited data available regarding gastrectomy. In a small subset of carefully selected patients, major gastric surgery can effectively relieve distressing vomiting from severe gastroparesis and improve quality of life in seriously affected patients in whom risk of subsequent renal failure is high and in whom life expectancy is poor. There are very few studies about outcomes after gastrectomy, but they were performed in patients with postsurgical-induced gastroparesis not diabetic gastroparesis. There is insufficient evidence in support of gastric surgery for the treatment of diabetic gastroparesis, and surgery is generally not recommended [43]. Symptoms may not be improved after gastrectomy due to concomitant small bowel denervation [44]. Additionally, patients with diabetic gastroparesis often have other comorbidities and are not ideal surgical candidates.

3.8   Miscellaneous Treatments

3.8.1   Psychological and Alternative Treatments

Anxiety and depression can be associated with gastroparesis, and consultation with a mental health provider may be helpful. Acupuncture, electroacupuncture, and acupressure stimulation of specific pressure points have been used for symptom relief. A meta-analysis of 14 randomized controlled studies showed that acupuncture had significantly improved dyspeptic symptoms (including nausea, vomiting, loss of appetite, and stomach fullness) compared with a control group, despite there being no difference in solid gastric emptying [45]. However, these studies were of low quality with a high risk of bias, and large-scale high-quality randomized clinical trials are needed.

3.8.2   Investigational Therapies

Camicinal, a motilin agonist, and relamorelin, a 5-HT4 receptor agonist, are investigational therapies for patients with diabetic gastroparesis [46–51]. There are also therapies under investigation that target pylorospasm and include pylorus stent placement, endoscopic pyloric myotomy, or laparoscopic pyloroplasty. In the future, stem cell therapies might be available.

3.9 Accelerated Emptying (Rapid Gastric Emptying)

In a subset of patients with diabetes, gastric emptying can be abnormally accelerated (also referred to a "dumping syndrome"). Symptoms are often difficult to distinguish from those with delayed gastric emptying. Patients with rapid gastric emptying can have poor postprandial glycemic control and postprandial upper abdominal symptoms such as abdominal discomfort, bloating, nausea, or vomiting. The bloating and abdominal discomfort can occur as a result of rapid filling, nutrient shifts, and small bowel distension rather than gastric distension [13]. Worsening symptoms with a prokinetic agent can be a sign of possible accelerated emptying. Gastric emptying studies will demonstrate accelerated emptying. For these patients, treatment includes avoidance of consuming fluids during and 30 min after meals as well as the addition of dietary fiber supplements (i.e., guar gum, pectin, locust bean gum) to delay gastric emptying. Treatment with GLP-1 agonists like exenatide, which are known to inhibit gastric emptying, may be required in addition to dietary maneuvers [54].

3.10 Conclusion

Diabetic gastroparesis is a serious complication of diabetes. The magnitude of delay in gastric emptying often does not correlate with the severity of symptoms. The main focus for management should be on control of hyperglycemia and dietary modifications. If symptoms are not responsive to dietary changes and glucose control, medication and surgical management may aid in symptom control.

References

1. Lyrenås EB, Olsson EH, Arvidsson UC, Orn TJ, Spjuth JH. Prevalence and determinants of solid and liquid gastric emptying in unstable type I diabetes. Relationship to postprandial blood glucose concentrations. Diabetes Care. 1997;20:413–8.
2. Horowitz M, Harding PE, Maddox AF, Wishart JM, Akkermans LM, Chatterton BE, et al. Gastric and oesophageal emptying in patients with type 2 (non-insulin-dependent) diabetes mellitus. Diabetologia. 1989;32:151–9.
3. Soykan I, Sivri B, Sarosiek I, Kiernan B, McCallum RW. Demography, clinical characteristics, psychological and abuse profiles, treatment, and long-term follow-up of patients with gastroparesis. Dig Dis Sci. 1998;43:2398–404.
4. Wang YR, Fisher RS, Parkman HP. Gastroparesis-related hospitalizations in the United States: trends, characteristics, and outcomes, 1995–2004. Am J Gastroenterol. 2008;103:313–22.
5. Bytzer P, Talley NJ. Dyspepsia. Ann Intern Med. 2001;134(9 Pt 2):815–22.
6. Manuscript A. NIH public access. Gastroenterology 2011;14:997–1003.
7. Wytiaz V, Homko C, Duffy F, Schey R, Parkman HP. Foods provoking and alleviating symptoms in gastroparesis: patient experiences. Dig Dis Sci. 2015;60:1052–8.
8. Halland M, Bharucha AE. Relationship between control of glycemia and gastric emptying disturbances in diabetes mellitus. Clin Gastroenterol Hepatol. 2016;14:929–36.
9. Gonlachanvit S, Hsu C-W, Boden GH, Knight LC, Maurer AH, Fisher RS, et al. Effect of altering gastric emptying on postprandial plasma glucose concentrations following a physiologic meal in type-II diabetic patients. Dig Dis Sci. 2003;48:488–97.
10. Bharucha AE, Kudva Y, Basu A, Camilleri M, Low PA, Vella A, et al. Relationship between glycemic control and gastric emptying in poorly controlled type 2 diabetes. Clin Gastroenterol Hepatol. 2015;13:466–76.e1.
11. Abell TL, Camilleri M, Donohoe K, Hasler WL, Lin HC, Maurer AH, et al. Consensus recommendations for gastric emptying scintigraphy: a joint report of the American neurogastroenterology and motility society and the society of nuclear medicine. Am J Gastroenterol. 2008;103:753–63.
12. Marathe CS, Rayner CK, Jones KL, Horowitz M. Relationships between gastric emptying, postprandial glycemia, and incretin hormones. Diabetes Care. 2013;36:1396–405.

13. Parkman HP, McCallum RW, Fass R. Clinical roundtable monograph treatment of patients with diabetic faculty. Postgraduate Institute for Medicine. 2009. www.gastroenterologyandhepatology.net/files/2013/05/gh1009_sup181.pdf. Accessed on 20 Sept 2016.

14. Bharucha AE, Batey-Schaefer B, Cleary PA, Murray JA, Cowie C, Lorenzi G, et al. Delayed gastric emptying is associated with early and long-term hyperglycemia in type 1 diabetes mellitus. Gastroenterology. 2015;149:330–9.

15. Kuo B, McCallum RW, Koch KL, Sitrin MD, Wo JM, Chey WD, et al. Comparison of gastric emptying of a nondigestible capsule to a radio-labelled meal in healthy and gastroparetic subjects. Aliment Pharmacol Ther. 2008;27:186–96.

16. Revicki DA, Camilleri M, Kuo B, Szarka LA, McCormack J, Parkman HP. Evaluating symptom outcomes in gastroparesis clinical trials: validity and responsiveness of the Gastroparesis Cardinal Symptom Index-Daily Diary (GCSI-DD). Neurogastroenterol Motil. 2012;24:456–63. e215–6

17. Sellin JH, Chang EB. Therapy insight: gastrointestinal complications of diabetes – pathophysiology and management. Nat Clin Pract Gastroenterol Hepatol. 2008;5:162–71.

18. Bujanda L. The effects of alcohol consumption upon the gastrointestinal tract. Am J Gastroenterol. 2000;95:3374–82.

19. Miller G, Palmer KR, Smith B, Ferrington C, Merrick MV. Smoking delays gastric emptying of solids. Gut. 1989;30:50–3.

20. Kuo P, Rayner CK, Jones KL, Horowitz M. Pathophysiology and management of diabetic gastropathy a guide for endocrinologists. Drugs. 2007;67:1671–87.

21. Perkel MS, Moore C, Hersh T, Davidson ED. Metoclopramide therapy in patients with delayed gastric emptying: a randomized, double-blind study. Dig Dis Sci. 1979;24:662–6.

22. Snape WJ, Battle WM, Schwartz SS, Braunstein SN, Goldstein HA, Alavi A. Metoclopramide to treat gastroparesis due to diabetes mellitus: a double-blind, controlled trial. Ann Intern Med. 1982;96:444–6.

23. McCallum RW, Ricci DA, Rakatansky H, Behar J, Rhodes JB, Salen G, et al. A multicenter placebo-controlled clinical trial of oral metoclopramide in diabetic gastroparesis. Diabetes Care. 1983;6:463–7.

24. Ricci DA, Saltzman MB, Meyer C, Callachan C, McCallum RW. Effect of metoclopramide in diabetic gastroparesis. J Clin Gastroenterol. 1985;7:25–32.

25. Rao AS, Camilleri M. Review article: metoclopramide and tardive dyskinesia. Aliment Pharmacol Ther. 2010;31:11–9.
26. Parkman HP, Carlson MR, Gonyer D. Metoclopramide nasal spray reduces symptoms of gastroparesis in women, but not men, with diabetes: results of a phase 2B randomized study. Clin Gastroenterol Hepatol. 2015;13:1256–63.e1.
27. Ray WA, Murray KT, Meredith S, Narasimhulu SS, Hall K, Stein CM. Oral erythromycin and the risk of sudden death from cardiac causes. N Engl J Med. 2004;9(351):1089–96.
28. Camilleri M. Clinical practice diabetic gastroparesis. N Engl J Med. 2007;356:820–9.
29. Parkman HP, Van Natta ML, Abell TL, McCallum RW, Sarosiek I, Nguyen L, et al. Effect of nortriptyline on symptoms of idiopathic gastroparesis: the NORIG randomized clinical trial. JAMA. 2013;310:2640–9.
30. Lacy BE, Crowell MD, Schettler-Duncan A, Mathis C, Pasricha PJ. The treatment of diabetic gastroparesis with botulinum toxin injection of the pylorus. Diabetes Care. 2004;27:2341–7.
31. Bromer MQ, Friedenberg F, Miller LS, Fisher RS, Swartz K, Parkman HP. Endoscopic pyloric injection of botulinum toxin A for the treatment of refractory gastroparesis. Gastrointest Endosc. 2005;61:833–9.
32. Arts J, van Gool S, Caenepeel P, Verbeke K, Janssens J, Tack J. Influence of intrapyloric botulinum toxin injection on gastric emptying and meal-related symptoms in gastroparesis patients. Aliment Pharmacol Ther. 2006;24:661–7.
33. Woodward MN, Spicer RD. Intrapyloric botulinum toxin injection improves gastric emptying. J Pediatr Gastroenterol Nutr. 2003;37:201–2.
34. Ezzeddine D, Jit R, Katz N, Gopalswamy N, Bhutani MS. Pyloric injection of botulinum toxin for treatment of diabetic gastroparesis. Gastrointest Endosc. 2002;55:920–3.
35. Friedenberg FK, Palit A, Parkman HP, Hanlon A, Nelson DB. Botulinum toxin A for the treatment of delayed gastric emptying. Am J Gastroenterol. 2008;103:416–23.
36. Arts J, Holvoet L, Caenepeel P, Bisschops R, Sifrim D, Verbeke K, et al. Clinical trial: a randomized-controlled crossover study of intrapyloric injection of botulinum toxin in gastroparesis. Aliment Pharmacol Ther. 2007;26:1251–8.
37. Camiller M, Parkman HP, Shafi MA, Abell TL, Gerson L. Clinical guideline: management of gastroparesis. Am J Gastroenterol. 2013;108:18–38.

38. Maple JT, Petersen BT, Baron TH, Gostout CJ, Wong Kee Song LM, Buttar NS. Direct percutaneous endoscopic jejunostomy: outcomes in 307 consecutive attempts. Am J Gastroenterol. 2005;100:2681–8.
39. Heckert J, Sankineni A, Hughes WB, Harbison S, Parkman H. Gastric electric stimulation for refractory gastroparesis: a prospective analysis of 151 patients at a single center. Dig Dis Sci. 2015;61:168–75.
40. O'Grady G, Egbuji JU, Du P, Cheng LK, Pullan AJ, Windsor JA. High-frequency gastric electrical stimulation for the treatment of gastroparesis: a meta-analysis. World J Surg. 2009;33:1693–701.
41. Toro JP, Lytle NW, Patel AD, Davis SS, Christie JA, Waring JP, et al. Efficacy of laparoscopic pyloroplasty for the treatment of gastroparesis. J Am Coll Surg. 2014;218:652–60.
42. Hibbard ML, Dunst CM, Swanström LL. Laparoscopic and endoscopic pyloroplasty for gastroparesis results in sustained symptom improvement. J Gastrointest Surg. 2011;15:1513–9.
43. Jones MP, Maganti K. A systematic review of surgical therapy for gastroparesis. Am J Gastroenterol. 2003;98:2122–9.
44. Camilleri M, Malagelada JR. Abnormal intestinal motility in diabetics with the gastroparesis syndrome. Eur J Clin Investig. 1984;14:420–7.
45. Yang M, Li X, Liu S, Li Z, Xue M, Gao D, et al. Meta-analysis of acupuncture for relieving non-organic dyspeptic symptoms suggestive of diabetic gastroparesis. BMC Complement Altern Med. 2013;13:311.
46. Hobson R, Farmer AD, Dewit OE, O'Donnell M, Hacquoil K, Robertson D, et al. The effects of camicinal, a novel motilin agonist, on gastro-esophageal function in healthy humans-a randomized placebo controlled trial. Neurogastroenterol Motil. 2015;27:1629–37.
47. Barshop K, Kuo B. The investigational drug camicinal for the treatment of gastroparesis. Expert Opin Investig Drugs. 2015;24:133–40.
48. Hellström P, Tack J, Johnson L, Hacquoil K, Barton M, Richards D, et al. The pharmacodynamics, safety, and pharmacokinetics of single doses of the motilin agonist, camicinal, in type 1 diabetes mellitus with slow gastric emptying. Br J Pharmacol. 2016;173:1768–77.
49. Camilleri M. Novel diet, drugs, and gastric interventions for gastroparesis. Clin Gastroenterol Hepatol. 2016;14:1072–80.

50. Camilleri M, Acosta A. Emerging treatments in neurogastroen-terology: relamorelin: a novel gastrocolokinetic synthetic ghrelin agonist. Neurogastroenterol Motil. 2015;27:324–32.
51. Acosta A, Camilleri M. Prokinetics in gastroparesis. Gastroenterol Clin North Am Elsevier Inc. 2015;44:97–111.
52. Sadiya A. Nutritional therapy for the management of diabetic gastroparesis: clinical review. Diabetes Metab Syndr Obes. 2012;5:329–35.
53. Alam U, Asghar O, Malik RA. Diabetic gastroparesis: therapeu-tic options. Diabetes Ther. 2010;1:32–43.
54. Drucker D, Nauck M. The incretin system: glucagon-like pep-tide-1 receptor agonists and dipeptidyl peptidase-4 inhibitors in type 2 diabetes. Lancet. 2006;368:1696–705.

Chapter 4
Small Intestine and Colon Complications in Patients with Diabetes

Ashish Sharma and Milena Gould Suarez

4.1 Introduction

Although gastrointestinal problems are extremely common in the general population, the incidence of certain gastrointestinal conditions such as diarrhea, small intestine bacterial overgrowth, constipation, and fecal incontinence is more common in diabetes mellitus (DM). Diabetic neuropathy plays a central role in their pathogenesis. Limited familiarity with these conditions associated with DM leads to delay in their recognition and appropriate management. In this chapter, the effects of DM on the small and large intestine, as well as the associated gastrointestinal problems, are discussed.

A. Sharma, MD (✉) • M.G. Suarez, MD
Department of Gastroenterology and Hepatology, Baylor College of Medicine, One Baylor Plaza, BCM-620, Houston, TX 77030, USA
e-mail: ashishdoc84@gmail.com; mgould@bcm.edu

J. Sellin (ed.), *Managing Gastrointestinal Complications of Diabetes*, DOI 10.1007/978-3-319-48662-8_4,
© Springer International Publishing AG 2017

4.2   Pathophysiology of Intestinal Dysfunction

Diabetic enteropathy encompasses small intestinal and colorectal dysfunctions such as diarrhea, constipation, and/or fecal incontinence. It is more commonly seen in patients with long-standing diabetes, especially in those with gastroparesis. Development of diabetic enteropathy is complex and multi-factorial. It involves both reversible and irreversible processes. Hypoglycemia and hyperglycemia have reversible effects on the metabolic and signaling pathways of enteric neurons and alter intestinal function in a manner that is potentially reversible with more effective glycemic control. However, gastrointestinal symptoms and complications do not always correlate with the duration of diabetes, glycemic control, or with the presence of autonomic neuropathy, which is often assumed to be the major cause of many gastrointestinal symptoms. Other pathophysiologic processes operative in diabetic enteropathy include enteric myopathy and neuropathy; however, causes of these abnormalities are unknown [1].

An intriguing and potentially important factor in diabetic enteropathy is the dysfunction of interstitial cells of Cajal (ICC). ICCs serve as pacemaker cells regulating intestinal motility and mediating peripheral nerve input to the gut. ICCs have many subtypes based on their anatomical location within the wall of the GI tract and are located in the myenteric plexus, circular or longitudinal muscle layer, deep muscular plexus, submucosa, or subserosa. Loss of ICC and an imbalance in the number of excitatory and inhibitory enteric nerves (autonomic neuropathy) are observed in gastric and intestinal regions in animal models of diabetes and in patients with the disease [2]. Decreased $\alpha2$-adrenergic input as a part of autonomic neuropathy causes altered adrenergic regulation of fluid and electrolyte transport [3]. Loss of ICC may be caused by reduced levels of trophic factors such as stem cell factor (SCF), which is normally produced by intestinal smooth muscle cells [4]. Decreased SCF production occurs when decreased insulin and/or insulin-like growth factor 1 signaling in patients with diabetes causes intestinal smooth muscle atrophy. Other potential etiologies of intestinal dysfunction in diabetic patients include ischemia and hypoxia from microvascular disease of the gastrointestinal tract, mitochondrial dysfunction, formation of irreversible advanced glycation end products, and peroxynitrite-mediated endothelial and enteric neuron damage [5].

Collectively, the effects of diabetes on several targets cause aberrations in gastrointestinal function and regulation. Loss of ICC, autonomic neuropathy, and imbalances in the number of excitatory and inhibitory enteric neurons can drastically alter complex motor functions such as peristalsis, reflexive relaxation, sphincter tone, vascular flow, and intestinal segmentation [5].

Small bowel and colonic diseases/complications associated with DM which will be discussed in this chapter include:

- Celiac disease
- Diabetic diarrhea
- Small intestine bacterial overgrowth (SIBO)
- Fecal incontinence
- Constipation
- Colon cancer

4.3   Celiac Disease

Celiac disease is an immune-mediated enteropathy in which dietary gluten leads to inflammation, villous atrophy of the small intestinal villi, and malabsorption. Celiac disease affects approximately 1 % of the US population; however, this risk is much higher in patients with type 1 diabetes mellitus (T1DM). Approximately 3–8 % of patients with T1DM have celiac disease [6]. In the vast majority of cases, the diagnosis of T1DM precedes that of celiac disease. Celiac disease and T1DM share human leukocyte antigen (HLA) and non-HLA susceptibility genes. A common environmental, microbial, or immunologic entity has been postulated but has not been fully elucidated. There is insufficient evidence for testing asymptomatic patients with T1DM for celiac disease; however, symptomatic patients with diarrhea/steatorrhea, weight loss, abdominal pain, and/or anemia should be screened [7, 8].

The pathology seen in celiac disease is due to initiation of innate and adaptive immune response resulting from permeation of α-gliadin (component of gluten found in wheat, rye, or barley) into lamina propria, as well as intraepithelial lymphocyte activation, that leads to an inflammatory infiltrate in the small bowel with villous destruction. This only happens in a genetically susceptible individual who possess HLA-DQ2 and/or HLA-DQ8 [9].

Clinical manifestations include abdominal pain, steatorrhea/diarrhea, weight loss, symptoms of anemia, or nutritional deficiencies. In young children with T1DM, sudden and perhaps paradoxical improvement in glycemic control due to malabsorption of nutrients should prompt screening for celiac disease. Celiac disease may have overlapping symptoms with irritable bowel syndrome (IBS) irrespective of the presence of DM; however, the current evidence regarding this relationship is conflicting [10, 11]. The most common dermatologic manifestation of celiac disease is dermatitis herpetiformis, a pruritic, erythematous blistering lesion located on extensor surfaces. The presence of this rash should also prompt testing for celiac disease.

Screening for celiac disease begins with serologic testing which includes a total immunoglobulin A (IgA) and tissue transglutaminase (TTG) IgA levels [12]. In individuals with low or absent IgA levels, the presence of deamidated gliadin peptide (DGP) IgG and/or TTG IgG antibodies may be a useful screening tool. In patients with >5 % probability of celiac disease (such as first-degree relatives of patients with celiac disease, patients with T1DM, autoimmune thyroid disease, and autoimmune liver disease) and negative serological status, upper endoscopy with duodenal bulb and distal duodenal biopsies should be obtained to confirm the diagnosis [13]. Endoscopic appearance of the duodenum may be abnormal with scalloping or flattening of folds. Duodenal biopsies may reveal a spectrum of changes including crypt hypertrophy, villous atrophy, and a lymphocytic inflammatory infiltrate [12]. Diagnostic algorithm for celiac disease is shown in Fig. 4.1 [13].

Elimination of dietary wheat, rye, and barley is the current therapy for celiac disease. Nutritional consultation and support groups may offer assistance in helping patients adhere to a gluten-free diet.

4.4   Diabetic Diarrhea

Diarrhea is a common complaint in DM. Diarrhea is defined as having more than three bowel movements per day, urgency, or loose, watery stools. According to one study, the adjusted odds ratio for diarrhea was 2.06 in patients with diabetes

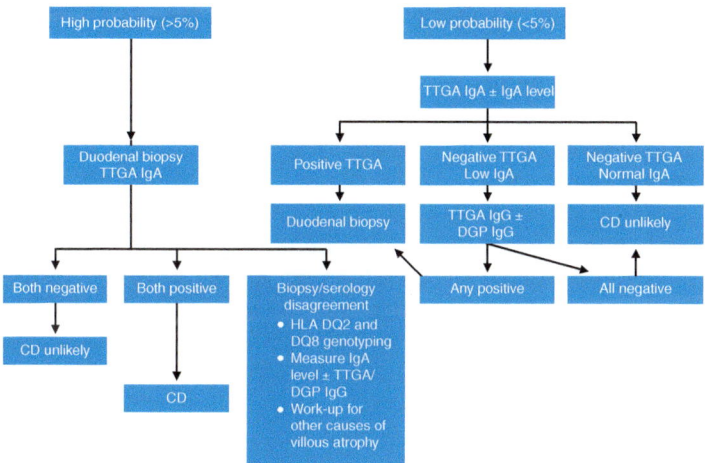

FIGURE 4.1 Celiac disease diagnostic testing algorithm. DGP, deamidated gliadin peptide; HLA, human leukocyte antigen; Ig, immunoglobulin; TTGA, tissue transglutaminase antibody (Reproduced from Rubio-Tapia [13] ©Nature)

when compared with controls, with a prevalence of diarrhea at 15.6 % [14].

Etiologies of diarrhea in diabetes are multifactorial and include rapid intestinal transit, drug-induced diarrhea, small intestine bacterial overgrowth, celiac disease, pancreatic exocrine insufficiency, dietary factors, anorectal dysfunction, fecal incontinence, and microscopic colitis [1]. Some of these etiologies are discussed separately later in this chapter.

A single or combination of multiple pathophysiological mechanisms may be responsible for diabetic diarrhea. Some of these mechanisms include diabetic enteropathy, decreased α2-adrenergic input, and intestinal dysmotility resulting in shortened or prolonged transit time. Medications (e.g., acarbose and miglitol) and dietary products (e.g., artificial sweeteners) can cause osmotic diarrhea. Metformin, which originates from a plant called goat's rue (*Galega officinalis*), increases the risk of diarrhea by threefold. This is related to decreased disaccharidase activity at brush border and increased serotonin levels [15]. Diarrhea can be early or late onset and is typically associated with dose escalation. Orlistat can cause fat malabsorption. Celiac disease and microscopic colitis are other common causes. Autoimmune pancreatitis can be associated with T1DM, resulting in pancreatic exocrine insufficiency and diarrhea [1, 16]. Diarrhea can be present when diabetes is a result of chronic pancreatitis (pancreatic diabetes [type 3C diabetes]). Autonomic neuropathy from poor glycemic control can affect anal sphincter function and rectal sensation, leading to fecal incontinence and diarrhea [1]. Autonomic neuropathy can also lead to orocecal transit time of <30 min, resulting in rapid intestinal transit and diarrhea [17]. It is important to differentiate whether diarrhea is caused by rapid intestinal transit vs. SIBO. Nuclear scintigraphy in combination with hydrogen breath tests can be helpful in this situation [17]. Newer technology such as wireless motility capsule may also be utilized [18]. This differentiation has key clinical implications with regard to the use of antimotility agents or antibiotics in a particular case. Figure 4.2 shows a diagnostic algorithm to help navigate a case of diabetic diarrhea [1].

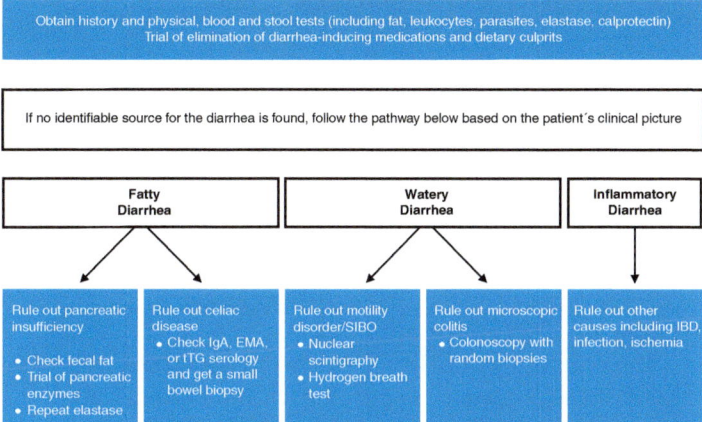

FIGURE 4.2 Diagnostic algorithm for diarrhea in the diabetic patient. This strategy can be used as a guide to workup diabetic diarrhea. EMA, epithelial membrane antigen; IBD, inflammatory bowel disease; SBBO, small bowel bacterial overgrowth; TTG, tissue transglutaminase (Reproduced with permission from Gould et al. [1] ©Springer)

Treatment of diabetic diarrhea starts with improved glycemic control. According to one study, patients with self-reported good glycemic control had a prevalence of 12.3 % of diarrhea symptoms, while those with poor control had a prevalence of 32.4 %. [14]. Identification of a specific etiology for diabetic diarrhea provides an opportunity for focused, effective therapy. Eliminating potential medicine or dietary triggers is important. Those with well-documented SIBO respond well to a rotating antibiotic regimen. Nonspecific therapy with loperamide generally controls rapid intestinal transit. More potent opiates (e.g., deodorized tincture of opium) are occasionally required. In patients who do not respond, clonidine, a α2-adrenergic agonist, can also treat idiopathic diarrhea [3]. However, it should be used with caution, given the potential for hypotension. Octreotide is another option in the diabetic patient with difficult-to-control diarrhea [19].

4.5   Small Intestine Bacterial Overgrowth

SIBO is characterized by alterations in the type and quantity of bacteria within the small intestine, resulting in significant changes in the microbiota of the small intestine causing gastrointestinal symptoms. In the general population, prevalence of symptomatic SIBO is estimated to be closer to 6 % [20]. However, the incidence of SIBO in patients with DM and diarrhea is much higher, approaching closer to 50 % in one study [20].

The pathology of SIBO is related to decreased acid in the stomach (acid decreases overall bacterial burden), abnormal gastrointestinal motility and slow transit (leads to stasis of intestinal contents and subsequent bacterial overgrowth), or structural abnormalities from surgeries, particularly blind loops, may also create reservoirs that enable overgrowth of bacteria. DM is known to cause gastroparesis and abnormal intestinal motility.

SIBO leads to carbohydrate malabsorption (due to disruption of intestinal brush border resulting in decreased disaccharidase activity), excessive gas production (from carbohydrate digestion by bacteria), and generation of inflammatory cytokines, short-chain fatty acids, and bile salt deconjugation. Due to bacterial deconjugation of bile salts, SIBO may lead to fat malabsorption and steatorrhea and subsequent deficiency of Vitamin A, D, E, and K [21]. Bile salt deconjugation may also lead to bile acid diarrhea due to direct secretory effect of bile acids on colonic mucosa and impaired enterohepatic reabsorption [22]. Anaerobic bacteria scavenge vitamin B12 leading to its deficiency. Figure 4.3 delineates the factors affecting development of SIBO [22, 23].

The typical symptoms of SIBO are nonspecific and include abdominal pain with bloating, gas, and diarrhea. Other frequently reported symptoms include flatulence, abdominal distension, and weakness. The symptoms are frequently vague and overlap with IBS-D. In patients with DM and the above symptoms, SIBO should be considered.

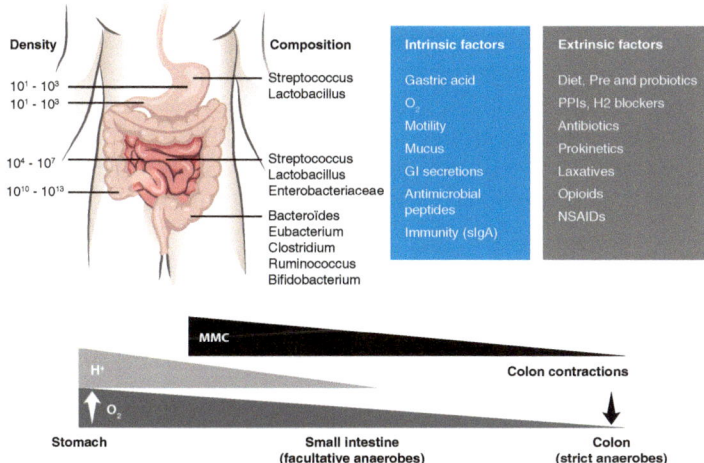

Quantification of bacteria from jejunal aspirate on EGD is the gold standard for diagnosis. A cutoff value of 100,000 CFU/mL is used. The test is costly, and it is cumbersome to handle specimen and difficult to culture intestinal bacteria, which makes it less practical. Other noninvasive tests such as glucose hydrogen breath test lack sensitivity, specificity, and accuracy when compared to bacterial quantification [24]. However, glucose hydrogen breath test when performed in combination with measurement of intestinal transit increases the accuracy of diagnosis. Given its practicality, empiric treatment with antibiotics is an acceptable alternative in most cases with suspected SIBO.

Management includes correction of the underlying conditions (such as impaired motility and poor glycemic control), correction of nutritional deficiencies (fat-soluble vitamins and vitamin B12), and use of antibiotics. Specifically for DM where intestinal motility may be impaired, good glycemic control and short-term use of prokinetics are advised. The most well studied and extensively used antibiotic is rifaximin for SIBO; however, its cost is a deterrent for routine use. Recurrence of SIBO is common and may respond to repeated courses of antibiotics. In refractory cases, patients may require continuous cycling of antibiotics to control symptoms. Judicious use of antibiotics is recommended. Table 4.1 delineates the antibiotic type and its duration for treatment of SIBO [25].

4.6   Fecal Incontinence

Fecal incontinence may affect up to 9 % of non-institutionalized US adults and is more common with older age [26, 27]. Specifically with diabetes, the odds ratio of developing fecal incontinence is 1.5 according to the largest cross-

TABLE 4.1 List of common antibiotics with their respective doses and duration of therapy used for treatment of small intestine bacterial overgrowth (SIBO)

Oral antibiotics	Dosage	Duration
Rifaximin	1,200–1,600 mg daily	10 days
Flagyl	250–500 mg BID to TID	7 days
Ciprofloxacin	250–500 mg BID	7–10 days
Tetracycline	250–500 mg QID	7 days
Doxycycline	100 mg BID	10 days
Augmentin	500/125 mg TID	7–10 days
Norfloxacin	400 mg BID	7 days

Adapted from Shah et al. [25] ©Wiley

sectional study to date based on the National Health and Nutrition Examination Survey (NHANES) database [26, 27]. Incontinence can be primary, caused by anorectal dysfunction, or secondary as a result of diarrhea. Fecal incontinence is related to autonomic neuropathy, impaired rectoanal reflex, and direct effect of glycemic control on internal anal sphincter [28, 29]. In a study evaluating anorectal sensory and motor function, researchers found that diabetic patients with fecal incontinence required a significantly larger volume to experience rectal sensation, which in turn leads to overflow incontinence [29]. Alternate etiologies such as damage to the internal anal sphincter from previous childbirth, surgery, or trauma should also be excluded. Fecal incontinence is distinct from stool seepage, producing soilage of undergarments that may result from hemorrhoids, enlarged skin tags, poor hygiene, fistula-in-ano, and rectal mucosal prolapse. Fecal incontinence manifests with low volume "diarrhea," and nocturnal symptoms are common.

Biofeedback therapy is effective in decreasing fecal soiling and increasing continence somewhat [29]. Although anal rectal dysfunction is attributable to autonomic neuropathy, evidence exists that acute changes in glucose can affect anorectal nerve function. In patients with DM, hyperglycemia affects external anal sphincter compliance and rectal compliance. These findings suggest improved glycemic control may improve fecal incontinence [28]. In addition, symptomatic treatment of diarrhea with loperamide or diphenoxylate may be a simple first step.

4.7   Constipation

Constipation is a common problem seen with long-standing DM. It is more common than in general population, where the incidence varies from 2 % to 30 % [30]. It affects 60 % of the patients with DM and is more common than diarrhea [14]. The prevalence of constipation is higher in women than men and is more prevalent among patients with diabetes who are taking medications that promote constipation such as calcium channel blockers [31].

Constipation is likely related to slow colonic transit caused by loss of ICC function and smooth muscle myopathy, although autonomic neuropathy and neuroendocrine imbalances might also contribute [5]. Diagnosis is clinical; however, a Sitz marker study and wireless motility capsule can be utilized to support the clinical diagnosis. Rare complications of constipation may include megacolon, intestinal-colonic pseudo-obstruction, stercoral ulcer, perforation, and overflow diarrhea [32].

There are no specific treatments for diabetes-associated constipation, although better glycemic control may be of some benefit. In most cases, patients are treated in the same way as those with idiopathic chronic constipation.

4.8   Colon Cancer

Colorectal cancer is the third most common cancer in men and the second in women [33]. Individuals with type 2 DM have an increased risk of colorectal cancer when compared with their nondiabetic counterparts [34]. With the global increase in type 2 DM, it is important to recognize this association. Shared risk factors for colorectal cancer and type 2 DM include obesity, sedentary lifestyle, and high-caloric diet. There has been a fairly consistent and moderate increased risk of colorectal cancer associated with type 2 DM vs. no diabetes and obesity vs. no obesity [35, 36]. This may be related to a progressive decrease in insulin sensitivity in diabetic patients leading to chronic compensatory hyperinsulinemia. Mechanistically, insulin may promote colorectal carcinogenesis through a cross talk with the insulin-like growth factor 1 (IGF-1) receptor, which stimulates epithelial cell proliferation and prolongs cell survival [36].

According to a recent large observational population-based cohort study, type 2 DM was associated with a 1.3-fold increased risk of colorectal cancer compared to the general population. Risk of colorectal cancer was significantly increased for patients with DM and recorded duration of obesity of 4 years or more [37]. Increased incidence of diabetes and obesity parallels the increased incidence and prevalence of colorectal cancer in the young patients (<50 years of age) in the last three decades [38].

At this time, there are no specific guidelines to perform colon cancer screening for younger patients with longer duration of type 2 DM and obesity. However, informing patients of this risk and counseling them about better glycemic control and weight are advised.

4.9   Conclusion

Diabetes can have a detrimental impact on the gastrointestinal tract by causing many symptoms ranging from diarrhea to constipation and, importantly, increasing a patient's risk of colon cancer. Physicians should have a high index of suspicion for diabetes-related small and large bowel diseases when treating a patient with DM and GI symptoms. In addition to glycemic control, dietary products and medications are important factors to consider in the causation of symptoms. Directing efforts at glycemic control are critical in helping patients with symptoms. Finally, evaluation for conditions such as celiac disease and colon cancer should be considered in the appropriate clinical setting.

References

1. Gould M, Sellin JH. Diabetic diarrhea. Curr Gastroenterol Rep. 2009;11:354–9.
2. He CL, Soffer EE, Ferris CD, Ferris CD, Walsh RM, Szurszewski JH, Farrugia G. Loss of interstitial cells of cajal and inhibitory innervation in insulin-dependent diabetes. Gastroenterology. 2001;121:427–34.
3. Fedorak RN, Field M, Chang EB. Treatment of diabetic diarrhea with clonidine. Ann Intern Med. 1985;102:197–9.

4. Horváth VJ, Vittal H, Lörincz A, Chen H, Almeida-Porada G, Redelman D, et al. Reduced stem cell factor links smooth myopathy and loss of interstitial cells of cajal in murine diabetic gastroparesis. Gastroenterology. 2006;130:759–70.
5. Sellin JH, Chang EB. Therapy insight: gastrointestinal complications of diabetes – pathophysiology and management. Nat Clin Pract Gastroenterol Hepatol. 2008;5:162–71.
6. Talal AH, Murray JA, Goeken JA, Sivitiz WI. Celiac disease in an adult population with insulin-dependent diabetes mellitus: use of endomysial antibody testing. Am J Gastroenterol. 1997;92:1280–4.
7. Sud S, Marcon M, Assor E, Palmert MR, Daneman D, Mahmud FH. 2010 Celiac disease and pediatric type 1 diabetes: diagnostic and treatment dilemmas. Int J Pediatr Endocrinol. 2010;2010:161285.
8. Chou R, Blazina I, Bougatsos C, et al. Screening for celiac disease: a systematic review for the U.S. Preventive Services Task Force. AHRQ Publication No. 14–05215-EF-1 May 2016.
9. Green PH, Cellier C. Celiac disease. N Engl J Med. 2007;357:1731–43.
10. Spiegel BM, DeRosa VP, Gralnek IM, Wang V, Dulai GS. Testing for celiac sprue in irritable bowel syndrome with predominant diarrhea: a cost-effectiveness analysis. Gastroenterology. 2004;126:1721–32.
11. Cash BD, Rubenstein JH, Young PE, Gentry A, Nojkov B, Lee D, et al. The prevalence of celiac disease among patients with nonconstipated irritable bowel syndrome is similar to controls. Gastroenterology. 2011;141:1187–93.
12. Van Der Windt DA, Jellema P, Mulder CJ, et al. Diagnostic testing for celiac disease among patients with abdominal symptoms: a systematic review. JAMA. 2010;303:1738–46.
13. Rubio-Tapia A, Hill ID, Kelly CP, Calderwood AH, Murray JA. American College of Gastroenterology. ACG clinical guidelines: diagnosis and management of celiac disease. Am J Gastroenterol. 2013;108:656–76.
14. Vinik A, Erbas T. Recognizing and treating diabetic autonomic neuropathy. Cleve Clin J Med. 2001;68:928–30. 932, 934–44
15. Bouchoucha M, Uzzan B, Cohen R. Metformin and digestive disorders. Diabetes Metab. 2011;37:90–6.
16. Tang Z, Sellin J. Malabsorption. In: Al B, editor. Nutritional care of the patient with gastrointestinal disease. Boca Raton: CRC Press Taylor and Francis Group; 2015.

17. Sellin JH, Hart R. Glucose malabsorption associated with rapid intestinal transit. Am J Gastroenterol. 1992;87:584–9.
18. Roland BC, Ciarleglio MM, Clarke JO, Semler JR, Tomakin E, Mullin GE, et al. Small intestinal transit time is delayed in small intestinal bacterial overgrowth. J Clin Gastroenterol. 2015;49:571–6.
19. Mourad FH, Gorard D, Thillainayagam AV, Colin-Jones D, Farthing MJ. Effective treatment of diabetic diarrhoea with somatostatin analogue, octreotide. Gut. 1992;33:1578–80.
20. Virally-Monod M, Tielmans D, Kevorkian JP, Bouhnik Y, Flourie B, Porokhov B, et al. Chronic diarrhoea and diabetes mellitus: prevalence of small intestinal bacterial overgrowth. Diabete Metab. 1998;24:530–6.
21. Dukowicz AC, Lacy BE, Levine GM. Small intestinal bacterial overgrowth: a comprehensive review. Gastroenterol Hepatol. 2007;3:112–22.
22. Bohm M, Siwiec RM, Wo JM. Diagnosis and management of small intestinal bacterial overgrowth. Nutr Clin Pract. 2013;28:289–99.
23. Simrén M, Barbara G, Flint HJ, Spiegel BMR, Spiller RC, Vanner S, et al. Intestinal microbiota in functional bowel disorders: a Rome foundation report. BMJ. 2013;62:159–76.
24. Corazza GR, Menozzi MG, Strocchi A, Rasciti L, Vaira D, Lecchini R, et al. The diagnosis of small bowel bacterial overgrowth. Reliability of jejunal culture and inadequacy of breath hydrogen testing. Gastroenterology. 1990;98:302–9.
25. Shah SC, Day LW, Somsouk M, Sewell JL. Meta-analysis: antibiotic therapy for small intestinal bacterial overgrowth. Aliment Pharmacol Ther. 2013;38:925–34.
26. Schiller LR, Santa Ana CA, Schmulen AC, Hendler RS, Harford WV, Fordtran JS. Pathogenesis of fecal incontinence in diabetes mellitus: evidence for internal-anal-sphincter dysfunction. N Engl J Med. 1982;307:1666–71.
27. Ditah I, Devaki P, Luma HN, Ditah C, Njei B, Jaiyeoba C, et al. Prevalence, trends, and risk factors for fecal incontinence in United States adults, 2005-2010. Clin Gastroenterol Hepatol. 2014;12:636–43.
28. Russo A, Botten R, Kong MF, Chapman IM, Fraser RJ, Horowitz M, et al. Effects of acute hyperglycaemia on anorectal motor and sensory function in diabetes mellitus. Diabet Med. 2004;21:176–82.
29. Wald A, Tunuguntla AK. Anorectal sensorimotor dysfunction in fecal incontinence and diabetes mellitus. Modification with biofeedback therapy. N Engl J Med. 1984;310:1282–7.

30. Andromanakos N, Skandalakis P, Troupis T, Filippou D. Constipation of anorectal outlet obstruction: pathophysiology, evaluation and management. J Gastroenterol Hepatol. 2006;21:638–46.

31. Maleki D, Locke 3rd GR, Camilleri M, Zinsmeister AR, Yawn BP, Leibson C, et al. Gastrointestinal tract symptoms among persons with diabetes mellitus in the community. Arch Intern Med. 2000;160:2808–16.

32. Krishnan B, Babu S, Walker J, Walker AB, Pappachan JM. Gastrointestinal complications of diabetes mellitus. World J Diabetes. 2013;4:51–63.

33. Ferlay J, Shin HR, Bray F, et al. Estimates of worldwide burden of cancer in 2008: GLOBOCAN 2008. Int J Cancer. 2010;127:2893–917.

34. Larsson SC, Orsini N, Wolk A. Diabetes mellitus and risk of colorectal cancer: a meta-analysis. J Natl Cancer Inst. 2005;97:1679–87.

35. Larsson SC, Wolk A. Obesity and colon and rectal cancer risk: a meta-analysis of prospective studies. Am J Clin Nutr. 2007;86:556–65.

36. Pollak M. The insulin and insulin-like growth factor receptor family in neoplasia: an update. Nat Rev Cancer. 2012;12:159–69.

37. Peeters PJ, Bazelier MT, Leufkens HG, et al. The risk of colorectal cancer in patients with type 2 diabetes: associations with treatment stage and obesity. Diabetes Care. 2015;38:495–502.

38. Siegel RL, Jemal A, Ward EM. Increase in incidence of colorectal cancer among young men and women in the United States. Cancer Epidemiol Biomark Prev. 2009;18:1695–8.

Chapter 5
Nonalcoholic Fatty Liver Disease

Aradhna Seth and Maya Balakrishnan

5.1   Introduction

Nonalcoholic fatty liver disease (NAFLD) is the main hepatic complication of obesity, insulin resistance, and diabetes and soon to become the leading cause for end-stage liver disease in the United States [1]. NAFLD is characterized by an accumulation of fat (steatosis) within >5 % of hepatocytes in the absence of secondary causes of hepatic steatosis. NAFLD is a spectrum of disease that ranges from steatosis (hepatic fat without significant hepatocellular injury) to nonalcoholic steatohepatitis (NASH; hepatic fat with hepatocellular injury) to advanced fibrosis and cirrhosis.

As a direct consequence of the obesity epidemic, NAFLD is the most common cause of chronic liver disease, while NASH is the second leading indication for liver transplantation [1]. NAFLD prevalence is estimated at 25 % globally [2] and up to 30 % in the United States [3–5]. Roughly 30 % of individuals with NAFLD also have NASH, the progressive subtype of NAFLD. Within the United States, NAFLD

A. Seth • M. Balakrishnan (✉)
Baylor College of Medicine, Section of Gastroenterology &
Hepatology, Houston, TX, USA
e-mail: maya.balakrishnan@bcm.edu

J. Sellin (ed.), *Managing Gastrointestinal Complications
of Diabetes*, DOI 10.1007/978-3-319-48662-8_5,
© Springer International Publishing AG 2017

prevalence varies among racial and ethnic subgroups, with the highest prevalence observed among Hispanic persons (estimated prevalence 27–29 %), followed by non-Hispanic whites (15–18 %) and non-Hispanic blacks (11–16 %) [6, 7]. NAFLD prevalence increases with age, and some studies suggest that NAFLD may be more prevalent among men compared to women [3, 5, 8].

Established risk factors for NAFLD are obesity, particularly central obesity, type 2 diabetes, hypertriglyceridemia, and the metabolic syndrome (Table 5.1) [9]. More recently recognized risk factors include polycystic ovarian syndrome and obstructive sleep apnea; the latter may contribute to NAFLD independent of obesity due to hypoxia perpetuating insulin resistance [10–12]. Patients with diabetes and NAFLD tend to have more aggressive diseases (vis-à-vis progression to cirrhosis and liver-related mortality) compared to those without diabetes [13]. NASH is estimated at 22 % among patients with diabetes, compared to 5 % of the general population [4, 14].

TABLE 5.1 Features of the metabolic syndrome. Metabolic syndrome is diagnosed in the presence of ≥3 features [52]

Cause	Method of evaluation
Central obesity	Waist circumference >102 cm in men
	Waist circumference >88 cm in women
Impaired fasting glucose	Fasting blood glucose >110 mg/dL
Hypertension	Systolic blood pressure >130 mmHg or diastolic blood pressure >85 mmHg
Hypertriglyceridemia	Triglycerides >150 mg/dL
Low HDL cholesterol	HDL <40 mg/dL in men, HDL <50 mg/dL in women

HDL high-density lipoprotein

5.2   Diagnosis

Current guidelines from the American Association of the Study of Liver Disease and the European Association for the Study of the Liver advise against routinely screening for NAFLD in the general population due to uncertainties surrounding diagnostic tests and treatment options [5, 15]. Thus, NAFLD is typically diagnosed following incidental detection of elevated aminotransferases or steatosis on abdominal imaging. NASH cirrhosis is often diagnosed incidentally after the discovery of cirrhosis.

Making a diagnosis of NAFLD requires demonstration of hepatic steatosis (by imaging or liver biopsy) and exclusion of secondary causes of hepatic steatosis and alternate causes of liver disease (Table 5.2). Clinical history, biochemical testing, and imaging findings are used in combination to diagnose NAFLD.

Patients with NAFLD may present with nonspecific symptoms such as fatigue or right upper quadrant pain but are generally asymptomatic. Physical exam may reveal hepatomegaly or signs of insulin resistance (dorsocervical hump or acanthosis nigricans). Women with NAFLD may have findings that raise suspicion for polycystic ovarian syndrome (i.e., history of irregular menses and/or infertility and hirsutism). Blood work may reveal elevated aspartate aminotransferase (AST) and alanine aminotransferase (ALT) two to three times the upper limit of normal, with aspartate transaminase (AST)/alanine transaminase (ALT) enzyme ratio <1. An AST/ALT ratio >1 may indicate the presence of cirrhosis. It is important to note that ALT and AST are often normal among patients with NAFLD and are not reliable indicators of the presence or severity of NAFLD [9, 16, 17].

If NAFLD is suspected in a patient with elevated aminotransferases, imaging should be done to evaluate for hepatic steatosis. Abdominal ultrasound, magnetic resonance imaging (MRI), and computed tomography (CT) scanning are the available imaging modalities. Abdominal ultrasound is the

TABLE 5.2 Secondary causes of hepatic steatosis and liver disease: suggested workup

Cause	Screening method	Abnormal values that should trigger further workup for alternative causes of liver disease
Alcohol	History	Heavy alcohol use defined as
		> 21 drinks/week for men
		>14 drinks/week for women for at least 2 years
Medications	Medication review for amiodarone, tamoxifen, corticosteroids, methotrexate, valproate, highly active antiretroviral therapy	Positive medication review
Infections	Hepatitis C antibody	Positive serology
	Hepatitis B surface antigen	
	Hepatitis B core antibody	
	HIV	
Wilson's disease (screen patients < 45 years)	Ceruloplasmin	Ceruloplasmin <20 mg/dL
Autoimmune hepatitis	Antinuclear antibody	Positive serology
	Smooth muscle antibody	
Iron overload	Ferritin	Transferrin saturation >45 % and ferritin >200 (premeuopausal woman) OR >300 (postmenopausal woman or man)
	Transferrin saturation	

first-line imaging test for steatosis. The advantages of ultrasound are that it is widely available, inexpensive, and noninvasive; the disadvantages are that it is operator dependent, limited by central obesity and overlying intestinal gas, and has a very low sensitivity detecting hepatic fat content <30% [18]. MRI is the most sensitive modality for detecting hepatic steatosis and can precisely map and quantify hepatic fat; however, its clinical use is restricted by limited availability, cost, and patient claustrophobia [19]. CT scan is the least favored option because it is the least sensitive for hepatic steatosis and is further limited by expense, radiation, and intravenous iodine contrast exposure [20]. None of these imaging techniques can be used to distinguish between the subtypes of NAFLD (simple steatosis vs. NASH) or to stage liver fibrosis.

A complete workup should be done to exclude alternative causes of hepatic steatosis and chronic liver disease as outlined in Table 5.2. The most frequent secondary causes of hepatic steatosis include hepatitis C infection (see Chap. 7), excessive alcohol intake, and a variety of medications such as amiodarone, tamoxifen, methotrexate, and steroids among others [5]. Autoantibodies (antinuclear antibody and anti-smooth muscle antibody) are positive up to 20 % of patients with NAFLD and are not associated with autoimmune hepatitis [21]. Serum ferritin is frequently elevated in the setting of NAFLD and may reflect inflammatory activity and/or insulin resistance. However, if positive autoantibodies or elevated ferritin are found, further diagnostic testing must be done to evaluate for autoimmune hepatitis and hemochromatosis, respectively, before concluding NAFLD. If there is diagnostic uncertainty, a liver biopsy should be performed.

Unfortunately, NASH may be diagnosed for the first time in a patient who has already developed cirrhosis. These patients are often described as having "cryptogenic cirrhosis." Patients with NASH cirrhosis will have typical physical exam and biochemical findings of cirrhosis. Imaging and liver biopsy are not useful for establishing NASH as the cause of cirrhosis. This is because advanced fibrosis results in permanent change in liver morphology with loss of steatosis and hepatocyte ballooning. When fatty acids accumulate causing lipotoxicity, the liver's protective mechanisms can become overwhelmed. Consequently, this activates several signaling pathways causing release of profibrotic cytokines and activation of hepatic stellate cells, both of which promote formation of fibrotic tissue [22]. Thus, imaging and liver histology will show findings of cirrhosis but will no longer demonstrate hepatic steatosis [23]. Instead, NASH is diagnosed based on exclusion of alternative causes of liver disease (Table 5.2) and medical history suggestive of a history of central obesity, features of metabolic syndrome, and/or type 2 diabetes.

5.3 NAFLD Subtypes, Natural History, and Prognosis

Compared to the general population, NAFLD is associated with excess mortality from three main causes in the following order: cardiovascular complications, (all-cause) malignancy, and liver disease [24, 25]. The two main subtypes of NAFLD are simple steatosis and NASH. Evaluation of liver histology is the only way to distinguish between NAFLD subtypes and is the basis for therapeutic decisions. Knowledge of the stage of fibrosis has important implications for prognosis. Liver disease-related mortality is primarily associated with NASH and with advanced fibrosis.

Simple steatosis (also known as nonalcoholic fatty liver) is characterized by the presence of steatosis without ballooned hepatocytes (which represents hepatocyte injury) or fibrosis. Mild inflammation may be present. Simple steatosis is associated with a very low risk of progressive liver disease and liver-related mortality. Because of the low risk of liver-related complications, the simple steatosis subtype does not require specific treatments for liver disease. Patients with simple steatosis are at an increased risk of cardiovascular complications compared to patients without NAFLD, particularly if there is concomitant diabetes. Therefore, cardiovascular risk factor reduction should be carefully pursued among patients with simple steatosis [5].

The presence of ballooned hepatocytes in addition to steatosis is the histologic feature diagnostic for NASH. Patients with NASH are at risk for progressive liver fibrosis and liver-related mortality, cardiovascular complications, and hepatocellular carcinoma (HCC) even in the absence of cirrhosis [26]. Liver fibrosis stage progresses at an estimated rate of one stage every 7 years [27]. Twenty percent of patients with NASH will eventually develop liver cirrhosis [9]. Therefore, management of patients with NASH should be geared toward reducing the risk of liver disease progression.

Fibrosis is the only histopathologic feature that predicts mortality [28, 29]. Fibrosis is staged using the Metavir scoring system and ranges from absent (stage 0) to cirrhosis (stage 4). Overall mortality is increased among patients with advanced fibrosis (stage 3–4) compared with no/early fibrosis (stage 0–2) irrespective of the extent of steatosis, ballooning, and inflammation [28]. The increased mortality seen among patients with advanced fibrosis is related to complications of liver disease, hepatocellular carcinoma, and possibly increased cardiovascular disease.

5.4   Indications for Liver Biopsy

Liver biopsy is vital to determining therapy and establishing prognosis of patients with NAFLD. Determination of a diagnosis of nonalcoholic steatohepatitis by liver biopsy is required prior to the initiation of liver specific treatments. In addition, liver biopsy allows for an assessment of hepatic fibrosis and provides important prognostic information regarding mortality. However, the cost, potential for complications, and invasive nature of liver biopsy limit its universal use among patients with NAFLD. Unfortunately, there are no guidelines with firm recommendations to guide the selection of candidates for liver biopsy, and clinicians have to rely on clinical risk factors to identify patients with NAFLD most at risk for progressing to NASH.

Insulin resistance is strongly associated with NASH. Metabolic syndrome, type 2 diabetes, and polycystic ovarian syndrome are associated with high risk of NASH on index liver biopsy [30]. In addition, risk of NASH increases with age (>45 years), hypertension, central obesity, dyslipidemia, the number of metabolic risk factors present, and those with a family history of diabetes [31].

Based on these observations, patients with NAFLD with features of the metabolic syndrome, insulin resistance, or type 2 diabetes should be considered for liver biopsy. Patients with persistently abnormal aminotransferases (>6 months) or clinical findings concerning for advanced fibrosis/cirrhosis should also be considered for liver biopsy [5, 9].

5.5   Noninvasive Methods for Predicting Fibrosis

Several noninvasive methods have been proposed for prediction of advanced fibrosis. These include clinical prediction models and liver elastography. While none are 100 % accurate, these tools are frequently incorporated into clinical practice to identify patients most at risk for advanced fibrosis and, therefore, targeted for liver biopsy. The best validated and most widely used clinical prediction model for advanced fibrosis is the NAFLD fibrosis score (NFS). The NFS is based on a formula consisting of routinely available clinical data (age, body mass index [BMI], presence of hyperglycemia, AST/ALT ratio, platelet count, and albumin) and is easily determined using an online calculator (http://nafldscore.com/). The formula provides an estimated stage of liver fibrosis for the individual patient, graded as F0–F4:

- F0: indicates the absence of fibrosis
- F1: perisinusoidal/portal fibrosis
- F2: perisinusoidal and portal/periportal fibrosis
- F3: septal or bridging fibrosis
- F4: indicating cirrhosis [25]

Loosely, the terms perisinusoidal, portal, and septal indicate the location of the fibrosis. F3 and F4 are considered stages of advanced fibrosis. A NFS score below −1.455 identifies patients at a low risk for advanced fibrosis (F3/F4) and has a negative predictive value of 88 %. An NFS above 0.676 identifies patients who are at a high risk for advanced fibrosis (F3/F4) with a positive predictive value of 82 %. An NFS score between −1.455 and 0.676 falls in an indeterminate range [32]. Depending on the study, 25–30 % of patients have an indeterminate score [32, 33]. Nevertheless, the intermediate category in addition to high risk has been shown to increase the likelihood of liver-related events and outcomes, including mortality and liver transplantation [34]. Therefore, when the NFS score is used to choose candidates for liver biopsy, an intermediate or high-risk score (NFS score >−1.455) is used as the threshold for liver biopsy.

Advances in imaging technology have yielded elastography techniques that can estimate hepatic fibrosis noninvasively. Elastography is based on the principle that liver stiffness increases with worsening liver fibrosis. Transient elastography (TE) and magnetic resonance elastography (MRE) are the two most extensively studied liver elastography methods for NAFLD. TE is an ultrasound-based elastography technique that uses mechanical vibrations to estimate elastography. TE can be performed in an office setting and has reasonably good accuracy for predicting advanced fibrosis/cirrhosis, but its use is limited among morbidly obese individuals [35]. MRE is more reliable and more accurate [36] than TE for estimating liver fibrosis but is not routinely available for clinical use.

5.6   Management

The risk of cardiovascular disease is increased across the entire NAFLD spectrum. Therefore, management of cardiovascular risk factors (hyperlipidemia, hypertension, and diabetes) is of foremost importance. When indicated, statins should be used for treatment of dyslipidemia. Statins are safe among patients with NAFLD (even in the setting of elevated liver enzymes) and are not associated with an increased risk of statin-induced hepatotoxicity [35]. All patients with NAFLD should be immunized against hepatitis A and hepatitis B and should be advised to avoid heavy alcohol intake (Table 5.2).

All patients should be directed to lose weight with the goal of achieving a normal BMI and waist circumference. Weight loss is associated with meaningful improvement in NASH histology. A recent prospective observational study among 293 patients with NASH demonstrated that 3–5 % weight loss is associated with improvement in steatosis, ≥7 % weight loss is associated with improvement in steatohepatitis (ballooning), and ≥10 % weight loss is associated with improvement in fibrosis and the highest likelihood of NASH resolution [37]. The challenge, however, is in motivating patients to achieve and maintain sufficient weight loss [38]. Cognitive behavioral therapy and frequent clinic visits counseling are possible strategies for encouraging weight loss. Bariatric surgery is associated with improvement in NAFLD, NASH, and fibrosis [39, 40]. Bariatric surgery should be considered among patients with severe obesity and complications but is not an established therapy for NASH at this time.

Exercise, independent of weight loss, is important for patients with NAFLD. At a minimum, the goal is for moderate-intensity exercise for ≥30 min daily at least 5 days per week, vigorous exercise for ≥20 min a day on 3 days a week, or some combination of both [41]. Exercise along these lines is associated with a significant reduction of hepatic fat [42]. Resistance training can improve muscle mass and thereby improve insulin resistance, a principle driver of NASH pathophysiology [42]. But the evidence for whether resistance training can improve hepatic fat is controversial. There is no evidence to show that any form of exercise improves hepatocyte ballooning or fibrosis. Patients with NAFLD, therefore, should be given recommendations to pursue regular aerobic exercise as outlined and may pursue resistance training as an additional intervention with the expectation that there might be improvements in insulin sensitivity and hepatic steatosis but not NASH or fibrosis.

The cornerstone of dietary recommendations is calorie restriction with the goal of weight loss. There is evidence to suggest that a Mediterranean diet is associated with reduction in hepatic steatosis and improvement in insulin sensitivity in the absence of weight loss [43]. However, there is not enough evidence to recommend a specific diet to patients with NAFLD [44]. Fructose intake is associated with greater risk of NAFLD, and "fast-food" diets consisting of high cholesterol, saturated fat, and fructose are associated with progressive fibrosis in animal models [45]. Therefore, intake of fructose and diets high in saturated fats and high cholesterol diet should be avoided.

In addition to lifestyle modifications and weight loss, liver-specific pharmacotherapy should be considered among patients with biopsy-proven NASH. Currently, there are no drugs approved by the US Food and Drug Administration (FDA) for the treatment of NASH, although vitamin E and pioglitazone are used off-label.

Vitamin E is an antioxidant that is recommended at a dose of 800 international units (IU) daily among nondiabetic non-cirrhotic patients with biopsy-proven NASH. Efficacy of vitamin E was initially demonstrated in the PIVENS trial where patients with NASH treated with 800 IU of vitamin E for 96 weeks had significant improvement in NASH histology as compared with placebo (43 % vs. 19 %, $P < 0.001$) [46]. These findings were confirmed in a subsequent trial [47]. The safety of long-term use of high-dose vitamin E in patients with NASH is still unknown. Data from outside of hepatology suggests that use of vitamin E at doses >400 IU daily is associated with a small increase in all-cause mortality, hemorrhagic stroke, and prostate cancer.

Thiazolidinediones (TZDs) are useful for treatment of NASH. Pioglitazone at a dose of 30–45 mg daily is recommended among non-cirrhotic patients with diabetes and biopsy-proven NASH. Pioglitazone was also examined in the PIVENS trial where it narrowly missed the primary end point but did show NASH resolution in 47 % of patients, as opposed to 21 % of placebo-treated patients

[46]. A later meta-analysis of four randomized controlled clinical trials (RCTs) demonstrated that TZDs improve steatosis, hepatocyte ballooning, and inflammation and may improve fibrosis [48]. More recently, in a single-center RCT among 101 patients with prediabetes or type 2 diabetes with NASH, pioglitazone was significantly associated with greater histologic improvement and NASH resolution when compared with placebo (histologic improvement: 58 % vs. 17 %, $P < 0.001$; NASH resolution: 51 % vs. 19 %, $P < 0.001$) [49]. Widespread use of pioglitazone has been limited due to concerns of associated weight gain (on average 3–5 kg) and concerns about the small but significant associated risks of heart failure, bladder cancer, and bone fractures among women [5]. Based on current evidence, however, pioglitazone is a treatment option for NASH in carefully selected patients with prediabetes and diabetes under close clinical monitoring for development of edema and weight gain and in conjunction with a hepatologist.

Obeticholic acid (OCA) and liraglutide are pipeline drugs that have shown promise for treatment of NASH in recent clinical trials. OCA is a synthetic bile acid and a farnesoid X nuclear receptor agonist. The FLINT trial, a recently completed phase III RCT, demonstrated that OCA-treated patients with NASH had significant improvement in NASH compared with placebo (45 % vs. 21 %, $P = 0.0002$). Importantly, patients treated with OCA also had more improvement in fibrosis and weight loss when compared to placebo. The most common adverse effect was pruritus and worsening dyslipidemia [50]. Liraglutide is a glucagon-like peptide-1 (GLP-1) receptor agonist approved for the treatment of type 2 diabetes and obesity. The LEAN trial, a recently completed phase II RCT, demonstrated that liraglutide-treated patients had greater resolution of NASH when compared to placebo (39 % vs. 9 %, $P = 0.019$) [51]. The drug was generally well tolerated, and adverse effects included mild to moderate diarrhea, constipation, and anorexia.

5.7   Summary

NAFLD is a highly prevalent condition with both hepatic and extrahepatic morbidity. Identifying the presence of NASH (a progressive NAFLD subtype) has therapeutic and prognostic implications. Currently, liver biopsy is the "gold standard" for diagnosis of NASH. Clinical markers that can be used to hone in on appropriate candidates to select for liver biopsy include the presence of metabolic syndrome features or an intermediate- to high-risk NAFLD fibrosis score. Cardiovascular risk reduction should be aggressively managed in all patients. Liver-specific therapies including vitamin E, pioglitazone, and/or consideration of clinical trials should be considered among patients with biopsy-proven NASH.

References

1. Wong RJ, Aguilar M, Cheung R, Perumpail RB, Harrison SA, Younossi ZM, Ahmed A. Nonalcoholic steatohepatitis is the second leading etiology of liver disease among adults awaiting liver transplantation in the United States. Gastroenterology. 2015;148:547–55.
2. Younossi ZM, Koenig AB, Abdelatif D, Fazel Y, Henry L, Wymer M. Global epidemiology of non-alcoholic fatty liver disease – meta-analytic assessment of prevalence. Incidence Outcomes Hepatol. 2015;64:73–84.
3. Vernon G, Baranova A, Younossi ZM. Systematic review: the epidemiology and natural history of non-alcoholic fatty liver disease and non-alcoholic steatohepatitis in adults. Aliment Pharmacol Ther. 2011;34:274–85.
4. Williams CD, Stengel J, l, Torres DM, Shaw J, Contreras M, et al. Prevalence of nonalcoholic fatty liver disease and nonalcoholic steatohepatitis among a largely middle-aged population utilizing ultrasound and liver biopsy: a prospective study. Gastroenterology. 2011;140:124–31.
5. Chalasani N, Younossi Z, Lavine JE, Diehl AM, Brunt EM, Cusi K, et al. The diagnosis and management of non-alcoholic fatty liver disease: practice guideline by the American Gastroenterological Association, American Association for the Study of Liver Diseases,

and American College of Gastroenterology. Gastroenterology. 2012;142:1592–609.

6. Lazo M, Hernaez R, Eberhardt MS, Bonekamp S, Kamel I, Guallar E, et al. Prevalence of nonalcoholic fatty liver disease in the United States: the Third National Health and Nutrition Examination Survey, 1988-1994. Am J Epidemiol. 2013;178:38–45.

7. Tota-Maharaj R, Blaha MJ, Zeb I, Katz R, Blankstein R, Blumenthal RS, et al. Ethnic and sex differences in fatty liver on cardiac computed tomography: the multi-ethnic study of atherosclerosis. Mayo Clin Proc. 2014;89:493–503.

8. Younossi ZM, Stepanova M, Afendy M, Fang Y, Younossi Y, Mir H, Srishord M. Changes in the prevalence of the most common causes of chronic liver diseases in the United States from 1988 to 2008. Clin Gastroenterol Hepatol. 2011;9:524–30.

9. Rinella ME. Nonalcoholic fatty liver disease: a systematic review. JAMA. 2015;313:2263–73.

10. Aron-Wisnewsky J, Minville C, Tordjman J, Levy P, Bouillot JL, Basdevant A, et al. Chronic intermittent hypoxia is a major trigger for non-alcoholic fatty liver disease in morbid obese. J Hepatol. 2012;56:225–33.

11. Corey KE, Misdraji J, Gelrud L, King LY, Zheng H, Malhotra A, Chung RT. Obstructive sleep apnea is associated with Nonalcoholic Steatohepatitis and Advanced Liver Histology. Dig Dis Sci. 2015;60:2523–8.

12. Musso G, Cassader M, Olivetti C, Rosina F, Carbone G, Gambino R. Association of obstructive sleep apnoea with the presence and severity of non-alcoholic fatty liver disease. A systematic review and meta-analysis. Obes Rev. 2013;14:417–31.

13. Younossi ZM, Gramlich T, Matteoni CA, Boparai N, McCullough AJ. Nonalcoholic fatty liver disease in patients with type 2 diabetes. Clin Gastroenterol Hepatol. 2004;2:262–5.

14. Marchesini G, Bugianesi E, Forlani G, Cerrelli F, Lenzi M, Manini R, et al. Nonalcoholic fatty liver, steatohepatitis, and the metabolic syndrome. Hepatology. 2003;37:917–23.

15. Ratziu V, Bellentani S, Cortez-Pinto H, Day C, Marchesini G. A position statement on NAFLD/NASH based on the EASL 2009 special conference. J Hepatol. 2010;53:372–84.

16. Browning JD, Szczepaniak LS, Dobbins R, Nuremberg P, Horton JD, Cohen JC, Grundy SM, et al. Prevalence of hepatic steatosis in an urban population in the United States: impact of ethnicity. Hepatology. 2004;40:1387–95.

17. Mofrad P, Contos MJ, Haque M, Sargeant C, Fisher RA, Luketic VA, Sterling RK, et al. Clinical and histologic spectrum of non-alcoholic fatty liver disease associated with normal ALT values. Hepatology. 2003;37:1286–92.

18. Hernaez R, Lazo M, Bonekamp S, Kamel I, Brancati FL, Guallar E, Clark JM. Diagnostic accuracy and reliability of ultrasonography for the detection of fatty liver: a meta-analysis. Hepatology. 2011;54:1082–90.

19. Schwenzer NF, Springer F, Schraml C, Stefan N, Machann J, Schick F. Non-invasive assessment and quantification of liver steatosis by ultrasound, computed tomography and magnetic resonance. J Hepatol. 2009;51:433–45.

20. Bohte AE, van Werven JR, Bipat S, Stoker J. The diagnostic accuracy of US, CT, MRI and 1H-MRS for the evaluation of hepatic steatosis compared with liver biopsy: a meta-analysis. Eur Radiol. 2011;21:87–97.

21. Adams LA, Lindor KD, Angulo P. The prevalence of autoantibodies and autoimmune hepatitis in patients with nonalcoholic fatty liver disease. Am J Gastroenterol. 2004;99:1316–20.

22. Feldman M, Friedman LS, Brandt LJ, editors. Sleisenger and Fordtran's gastrointestinal and liver disease. Philadelphia: Saunders/Elsevier; 2016.

23. Poonawala A, Nair SP, Thuluvath PJ. Prevalence of obesity and diabetes in patients with cryptogenic cirrhosis: a case-control study. Hepatology. 2000;32:689–92.

24. Ong JP, Aggarwal A, Krieger D, Easley KA, Karafa MT, Van Lente F, et al. Correlation between ammonia levels and the severity of hepatic encephalopathy. Am J Med. 2003;114:188–93.

25. Adams LA, Lymp JF, St Sauver J, Sanderson SO, Lindor KD, Feldstein A, Angulo P. The natural history of nonalcoholic fatty liver disease: a population-based cohort study. Gastroenterology. 2005;129:113–21.

26. Piscaglia F, Svegliati-Baroni G, Barchetti A, Pecorelli A, Marinelli S, Tiribelli C, Bellentani S. Clinical patterns of hepatocellular carcinoma (hcc) in non alcoholic fatty liver disease (NAFLD): a multicenter prospective study. Hepatology. 2015;63:827–38.

27. Singh S, Allen AM, Wang Z, Prokop LJ, Murad MH, Loomba R. Fibrosis progression in nonalcoholic fatty liver vs nonalcoholic steatohepatitis: a systematic review and meta-analysis of paired-biopsy studies. Clin Gastroenterol Hepatol. 2015;13:643–54.

28. Angulo P, Kleiner DE, Dam-Larsen S, Adams LA, Bjornsson ES, Charatcharoenwitthaya P, et al. Liver fibrosis, but no other histologic features, is associated with long-term outcomes of patients with nonalcoholic fatty liver disease. Gastroenterology. 2015;149:389–97.

29. Ekstedt M, Hagstrom H, Nasr P, Fredrikson M, Stal P, Kechagias S, Hultcrantz R. Fibrosis stage is the strongest predictor for disease-specific mortality in NAFLD after up to 33 years of follow-up. Hepatology. 2015;61:1547–54.

30. Ahmed A, Wong RJ, Harrison SA. Nonalcoholic fatty liver disease review: diagnosis, treatment, and outcomes. Clin Gastroenterol Hepatol. 2015;13:2063–70.

31. Dixon JB, Bhathal PS, O'Brien PE. Nonalcoholic fatty liver disease: predictors of nonalcoholic steatohepatitis and liver fibrosis in the severely obese. Gastroenterology. 2001;121:91–100.

32. Angulo P, Hui JM, Marchesini G, Bugianesi E, George J, Farrell GC, et al. The NAFLD fibrosis score: a noninvasive system that identifies liver fibrosis in patients with NAFLD. Hepatology. 2007;45:846–54.

33. Ruffillo G, Fassio E, Alvarez E, Landeira G, Longo C, Dominguez N, Gualano G. Comparison of NAFLD fibrosis score and BARD score in predicting fibrosis in nonalcoholic fatty liver disease. J Hepatol. 2011;54:160–3.

34. Angulo P, Bugianesi E, Bjornsson ES, Charatcharoenwitthaya P, Mills PR, Barrera F, et al. Simple noninvasive systems predict long-term outcomes of patients with nonalcoholic fatty liver disease. Gastroenterology. 2013;145:782–9.

35. Sandrin L, Fourquet B, Hasquenoph JM, Yon S, Fournier C, Mal F, et al. Transient elastography: a new noninvasive method for assessment of hepatic fibrosis. Ultrasound Med Biol. 2003;29:1705–13.

36. Huwart L, Peeters F, Sinkus R, Annet L, Salameh N, ter Beek LC, et al. Liver fibrosis: non-invasive assessment with MR elastography. NMR Biomed. 2006;19:173–9.

37. Vilar-Gomez E, Martinez-Perez Y, Calzadilla-Bertot L, Torres-Gonzalez A, Gra-Oramas B, Gonzalez-Fabian L, et al. Weight loss via lifestyle modification significantly reduces features of nonalcoholic steatohepatitis. Gastroenterology. 2015;149:367–78.

38. Centis E, Moscatiello S, Bugianesi E, Bellentani S, Fracanzani AL, Calugi S, et al. Stage of change and motivation to healthier

lifestyle in non-alcoholic fatty liver disease. J Hepatol. 2013;58:771–7.

39. Mathurin P, Hollebecque A, Arnalsteen L, Buob D, Leteurtre E, Caiazzo R, et al. Prospective study of the long-term effects of bariatric surgery on liver injury in patients without advanced disease. Gastroenterology. 2009;137:532–40.

40. Taitano AA, Markow M, Finan JE, Wheeler DE, Gonzalvo JP, Murr MM. Bariatric surgery improves histological features of nonalcoholic fatty liver disease and liver fibrosis. J Gastrointest Surg. 2015;19:429–36.

41. World Health Organization. Global recommendations on physical activity for health. World Health Organisation: Geneva; 2010. www.who.int/dietphysicalactivity/factsheet_recommendations/en/. Accessed 19 July 2016.

42. Keating SE, George J, Johnson NA. The benefits of exercise for patients with non-alcoholic fatty liver disease. Expert Rev Gastroenterol Hepatol. 2015;9:1247–50.

43. Ryan MC, Itsiopoulos C, Thodis T, Ward G, Trost N, Hofferberth S, et al. The Mediterranean diet improves hepatic steatosis and insulin sensitivity in individuals with non-alcoholic fatty liver disease. J Hepatol. 2013;59:138–43.

44. Zivkovic AM, German JB, Sanyal AJ. Comparative review of diets for the metabolic syndrome: implications for nonalcoholic fatty liver disease. Am J Clin Nutr. 2007;86:285–300.

45. Charlton M, Krishnan A, Viker K, Sanderson S, Cazanave S, McConico A, et al. Fast food diet mouse: novel small animal model of NASH with ballooning, progressive fibrosis, and high physiological fidelity to the human condition. Am J Physiol Gastrointest Liver Physiol. 2011;301:G825–34.

46. Sanyal AJ, Chalasani N, Kowdley KV, McCullough A, Diehl AM, Bass NM, et al. Pioglitazone, vitamin E, or placebo for nonalcoholic steatohepatitis. N Engl J Med. 2010;362:1675–85.

47. Lavine JE, Schwimmer JB, Van Natta ML, Molleston JP, Murray KF, Rosenthal P, et al. Effect of vitamin E or metformin for treatment of nonalcoholic fatty liver disease in children and adolescents: the TONIC randomized controlled trial. JAMA. 2011;305:1659–68.

48. Boettcher E, Csako G, Pucino F, Wesley R, Loomba R. Meta-analysis: pioglitazone improves liver histology and fibrosis in patients with non-alcoholic steatohepatitis. Aliment Pharmacol Ther. 2012;35:66–75.

49. Cusi K, Orsak B, Bril F, Lomonaco R, Hecht J, Ortiz-Lopez C, et al. Long-term pioglitazone treatment for patients with nonalcoholic steatohepatitis and prediabetes or type 2 diabetes mellitus: a randomized, controlled trial. Ann Intern Med 2016; [Epub ahead of print].

50. Neuschwander-Tetri BA, Loomba R, Sanyal AJ, Lavine JE, Van Natta ML, Abdelmalek MF, et al. Farnesoid X nuclear receptor ligand obeticholic acid for non-cirrhotic, non-alcoholic steatohepatitis (FLINT): a multicentre, randomised, placebo-controlled trial. Lancet. 2014;385:956–65.

51. Armstrong MJ, Gaunt P, Aithal GP, Barton D, Hull D, Parker R, et al. Liraglutide safety and efficacy in patients with non-alcoholic steatohepatitis (LEAN): a multicentre, double-blind, randomised, placebo-controlled phase 2 study. Lancet. 2015;387:679–90.

52. National Cholesterol Education Program (NCEP) Expert Panel on Detection, Evaluation, and Treatment of High Blood Cholesterol in Adults (Adult Treatment Panel III). Third Report of the National Cholesterol Education Program (NCEP) Expert Panel on Detection, Evaluation, and Treatment of High Blood Cholesterol in Adults (Adult Treatment Panel III) final report. Circulation 2002;106:3143–421.

Chapter 6
Nonalcoholic Fatty Liver Disease and Hepatocellular Carcinoma

Randy Chung and Sahil Mittal

6.1 Introduction

Nonalcoholic fatty liver disease (NAFLD) has emerged as the most common etiology of chronic liver disease in the United States and other developed countries (see Chap. 5) [1]. NAFLD encompasses a broad clinicopathologic spectrum of disease ranging from simple hepatic steatosis to nonalcoholic steatohepatitis (NASH). Patients with NAFLD, especially NASH, are at risk for developing cirrhosis and its associated complications, including hepatocellular carcinoma (HCC). With the increasing prevalence of NAFLD closely linked to the growing epidemics of diabetes mellitus and obesity, NAFLD-related HCC is expected to rise.

R. Chung
University of Texas Southwestern, Dallas, TX, USA
e-mail: randy.chung@phhs.org

S. Mittal (✉)
Kelsey-Sebold Clinic, Houston, TX, USA
e-mail: smittal@bcm.edu

J. Sellin (ed.), *Managing Gastrointestinal Complications of Diabetes*, DOI 10.1007/978-3-319-48662-8_6,
© Springer International Publishing AG 2017

83

6.2 Association Between Nonalcoholic Fatty Liver Disease and Hepatocellular Carcinoma

HCC is the most common primary malignancy of the liver and globally is the fifth most common cancer [2]. The majority of HCC cases occur in less developed countries such as East Asia and sub-Saharan Africa, though the incidences in these countries are decreasing. On the other hand, the incidence of HCC has been on the rise in developed countries, including the United States, which has seen a threefold increase between 1975 and 2007 [3]. Chronic hepatitis C virus (HCV) accounts for about half of this increase [2]. However, 15–50 % of new cases of HCC are labeled as cryptogenic or idiopathic, which suggests that other risk factors are likely playing a role [4].

NASH has been proposed as the underlying cause of most cases of cryptogenic cirrhosis. Multiple retrospective studies have compared patients who develop HCC in the setting of cryptogenic cirrhosis and patients with HCC from viral- or alcoholic-related cirrhosis. Analysis from this comparison has confirmed that features associated with NASH, including diabetes, insulin resistance, obesity, and dyslipidemia, were all significantly associated with cryptogenic cirrhosis [5]. Patients with cryptogenic cirrhosis have a similar prevalence of diabetes and obesity to that of patients with NASH and a significantly higher prevalence than in patients with cirrhosis from viral and autoimmune disease [6]. In a Korean study, HCC associated with cryptogenic cirrhosis also correlated with increased age, increased occurrence of the metabolic syndrome, and less aggressive tumor characteristics, which are all features that have been associated with NASH-related HCC [7]. A large proportion of cryptogenic cirrhosis, therefore, likely represents end-stage NASH.

6.3   Increased Risk of Hepatocellular Carcinoma in Nonalcoholic Fatty Liver Disease

Epidemiologic evidence supports an association between NASH and a significant increase in risk of HCC that seems to be predominantly limited to individuals with cirrhosis. In a large systematic review published in 2012, NAFLD or NASH cohorts with few or no cirrhosis cases demonstrated a minimal HCC risk with cumulative HCC mortality between 0 % and 3 % over study periods of up to two decades [8]. In contrast, consistently increased risk was observed in NASH-cirrhosis cohorts with cumulative incidence between 2.4 % over 7 years and 12.8 % over 3 years [8]. The risk of HCC was substantially lower among patients with NASH than in patients with viral hepatitis [8]. However, given the high and increasing prevalence of NAFLD, even a small increase in risk of HCC has the potential to transform into a huge case burden of HCC.

Fatty liver may also affect the risk of HCC in other liver diseases. In patients with HCV, the risk of HCC has been shown to be two- to threefold greater in the presence of hepatic steatosis than in those without steatosis [9]. However, opposite trends have been observed for steatosis and HCC risk in patients with chronic hepatitis B. Steatosis has been associated with decreased viral loads in chronic hepatitis B [10].

6.4   Risk Factors for Hepatocellular Carcinoma in Nonalcoholic Fatty Liver Disease

Regardless of underlying liver disease, cirrhosis remains the single most important risk factor for HCC and is present in about 80–90 % of patients with HCC [11]. Presence of cirrhosis or advanced fibrosis is one of the strongest predictors for development of HCC in NAFLD.

Numerous studies have consistently reported higher prevalence of diabetes mellitus and obesity among NASH patients with HCC than among NASH patients without HCC. Large population-based cohort studies from Europe have demonstrated a 1.86-fold to fourfold increase in risk of HCC among patients with diabetes [12]. Obesity, which is well established as a significant risk factor for the development of various malignancies, is associated with a 1.5-fold to fourfold increased risk for development of HCC [13]. Therefore, the excess risk of HCC in NAFLD is explained by both the increased risk for NAFLD itself with subsequent progression to NASH and the independent carcinogenic potential of diabetes and obesity [11].

Emerging evidence suggests that excess sinusoidal iron deposition in NASH may play a role in liver injury as well as its progression to HCC [14, 15]. A retrospective study from Italy showed that high hepatic iron deposition was a risk factor for HCC among patients with NASH-related cirrhosis compared with age- and gender-matched NASH controls with cirrhosis but without HCC [16].

In addition to diabetes and obesity, PNPLA3 single-nucleotide polymorphism (SNP) is strongly linked with development of NASH. The encoded protein of this gene may be involved in the balance of energy usage and liver fat accumulation. A recent meta-analysis showed that PNPLA3 was associated with increased risk of HCC in patients with cirrhosis, but this increased risk of HCC was limited to patients with NASH- or alcohol-related cirrhosis compared with cirrhosis with other etiologies [17].

6.5   Hepatocellular Carcinoma in Absence of Cirrhosis

Cirrhosis is considered a precancerous condition for the majority of cases of HCC, with studies in hepatitis B virus and HCV reporting more than 90 % of HCC cases occurring in the setting of cirrhosis or at least advanced fibrosis. However, there is growing literature reporting that HCC can develop in patients with NASH but without cirrhosis. In a study of a national cohort of 1,500 veterans diagnosed with HCC, 35 % of NAFLD-related HCC and 19 % of HCC with metabolic syndrome did not have evidence of cirrhosis at the time of HCC diagnosis, compared with 10 % of those with HCV- or alcohol-related HCC [18]. A single-center study among HCC patients undergoing curative resection evaluated explant specimens and found significantly lower prevalence of cirrhosis among NASH-HCC than HCV- or alcohol-related HCC (73 % vs. 94 %, $P < 0.05$) [19]. Therefore, the proportion of patients with NASH who progress to HCC without cirrhosis is much higher compared to HCV- or alcohol-related HCC. However, the mechanisms responsible for this progression of non-cirrhotic NAFLD to HCC are not fully understood.

6.6   Clinical Features of Nonalcoholic Fatty Liver Disease-Related Hepatocellular Carcinoma

In contrast to patients with HCC from other causes, patients with NAFLD-related HCC tend to be older and have more metabolic comorbidities but less severe liver dysfunction [20]. Tumor markers are also differentially expressed; levels of alpha-fetoprotein are raised less frequently, and levels of des-gamma carboxythrombin are raised more frequently in patients with NAFLD-related HCC than in HCC as a result of other liver diseases [21]. Tumors are typically larger in size and more often well differentiated compared to HCC-related viral hepatitis. However, the overall 5-year survival remains similar between patients with cirrhosis who have NAFLD-related HCC or chronic HCV-related HCC [21].

6.7   Pathophysiology of Hepatocellular Carcinoma in Nonalcoholic Fatty Liver Disease

The exact mechanisms responsible for the development of HCC in NASH remain unclear. Available evidence suggests that the similar pathophysiologic mechanisms behind the development of NASH related to insulin resistance and the subsequent inflammatory cascade likely also contribute to the carcinogenic potential of NASH. Oxidative stress and release of reactive oxygen species have also been implicated in the development of HCC through steatosis, hepatic inflammation, hepatocyte proliferation, and direct induction of cancer-promoting mutations [22]. Insulin resistance related to diabetes, obesity, or metabolic syndrome is thought to stimulate release of multiple pro-inflammatory cytokines which subsequently leads to hepatocyte death, compensatory proliferation, and ultimately carcinogenesis [23, 24]. Further evidence comes from epidemiologic evidence showing that treatment of diabetes with an insulin sensitizer, such as metformin, resulted in a significantly reduced risk of HCC compared with no treatment, treatment with insulin, or insulin secretagogues [25].

6.8   Clinical Implications

Complications of NAFLD are expected to increase with the continuing epidemics of diabetes and obesity. Although patients with NAFLD have an increased risk of HCC compared with the general population, current epidemiological data do not support routine HCC screening for NAFLD or NASH patients in the absence of cirrhosis. Once the diagnosis of cirrhosis is made, however, screening for HCC should be pursued (Table 6.1).

While additional research is necessary on the risk factors of HCC in NAFLD, available evidence already suggests that

TABLE 6.I Recommendations for screening for hepatocellular carcinoma (HCC) in nonalcoholic fatty liver disease (NAFLD)

Clinical indication	Strength of evidence for increased risk of HCC	Recommendation
NAFLD with cirrhosis	Strong	Screen for HCC with liver ultrasound every 6 months
NAFLD without cirrhosis	Emerging evidence	HCC screening not recommended at present

diabetes, insulin resistance, and obesity likely play an important role in carcinogenesis. The epidemiological association indicates that absence of these conditions is associated with a reduction in HCC risk. What remains less clear is whether treatment will result in a benefit. However, it is reasonable to seek and maximize management of concomitant metabolic conditions in patients with NAFLD with the hope of reducing the risk of progression to HCC.

References

1. Adams LA, Lindor KD. Nonalcoholic fatty liver disease. Ann Epidemiol. 2007;17:863–9.
2. Gomaa AI, Khan SA, Toledano MB, Waked I, Taylor-Robinson SD. Hepatocellular carcinoma: epidemiology, risk factors, and pathogenesis. World J Gastroenterol. 2008;14:4300–8.
3. El-Serag HB, Davila JA, Petersen NJ, McGlynn KA. The continuing increase in the incidence of hepatocellular carcinoma in the United States: an update. Ann Intern Med. 2003;139:817–23.
4. El-Serag HB. Epidemiology of hepatocellular carcinoma in USA. Hepatol Res. 2007;37(Suppl 2):S88–94.
5. Bugianesi E, Leone N, Vanni E, Marchesini G, Brunello F, Carucci P, et al. Expanding the natural history of nonalcoholic steatohepatitis: from cryptogenic cirrhosis to hepatocellular carcinoma. Gastroenterology. 2002;123:134–40.

6. Caldwell SH, Oelsner DH, Iezzone JC, Hespenheide EE, Battle EH, Driscoll CJ. Cryptogenic cirrhosis: clinical characterization and risk factors for underlying disease. Hepatology. 1999;29:664–9.

7. Lee SS, Jeong SH, Byoun YS, Chung SM, Seong MH, Sohn HR, et al. Clinical features and outcome of cryptogenic hepatocellular carcinoma compared to those of viral and alcoholic hepatocellular carcinoma. BMC Cancer. 2013;13:335.

8. White DL, Kanwal F, El-Serag HB. Non-alcoholic fatty liver disease and hepatocellular cancer: a systematic review. Clin Gastroenterol Hepatol. 2012;10:1342–59.

9. Sanyal AJ, Banas C, Sargeant C, et al. Similarities and differences in outcomes of cirrhosis due to nonalcoholic steatohepatitis and hepatitis C. Hepatology. 2006;43:682–9.

10. Machado MV, Oliveira AG, Cortez-Pinto H. Hepatic steatosis in hepatitis B virus infected patients: meta-analysis of risk factors and comparison with hepatitis C infected patients. J Gatroenterol Hepatol. 2011;2006:1361–7.

11. Bugianesi E. Non-alcoholic steatohepatitis and cancer. Clin Liver Dis. 2007;11:191–207.

12. Adami HO, Chow WH, Nyren O, Berne C, Linet MS, Ekbom A, et al. Excess risk of primary liver cancer in patients with diabetes mellitus. J Natl Cancer Inst. 1996;88:1472–7.

13. Calle EE, Rodriguez C, Walker-Thurmond K, Thun MJ. Overweight, obesity, and mortality from cancer in a prospectively studied cohort of U.S. adults. N Engl J Med. 2003;348:1625–38.

14. Pietrangelo A. Iron in NASH, chronic liver diseases and HCC: how much iron is too much? J Hepatol. 2009;50:249–51.

15. George DK, Goldwurm S, MacDonald GA, Cowley LL, Walker NI, Ward PJ, et al. Increased hepatic iron concentration in non-alcoholic steatohepatitis is associated with increased fibrosis. Gastroenterology. 1998;114:311–8.

16. Sorrentino P, D'Angelo S, Ferbo U, Micheli P, Braciagliano A, Vechione R. Liver iron excess in patients with hepatocellular carcinoma developed on non-alcoholic steato-hepatitis. J Hepatol. 2009;50:351–7.

17. Singal AG, Manjunath H, Yopp AC, Beg MS, Marrero JA, Gopal P, et al. The effect of PNPLA3 on fibrosis progression and development of hepatocellular carcinoma: a meta-analysis. Am J Gastroenterol. 2014;109:325–34.

18. El-Serag H, Mittal S, Kanwal F, Duan Z, Sada Y, Temple S, et al. HCC in the absence of cirrhosis in United States veterans: an emerging disease entity associated with features of metabolic syndrome. Gastroenterol. 2014;146:S-917.

19. Reddy SK, Steel JL, Chen HW, DeMateo DJ, Cardinal J, Behari J, et al. Outcomes of curative treatment for hepatocellular cancer in nonalcoholic steatohepatitis versus hepatitis C and alcoholic liver disease. Hepatology. 2012;55:1809–19.

20. Duan XY, Qio L, Fan JG. Clinical features of nonalcoholic fatty liver disease-associated hepatocellular carcinoma. Hepatobiliary Pancreat Dis Int. 2012;11:18–27.

21. Tokushige K, Hashimoto E, Horie Y, Taniai M, Higuchi S. Hepatocellular carcinoma in Japanese patients with nonalcoholic fatty liver disease, alcoholic liver disease, and chronic liver disease of unknown etiology: report of the nationwide survey. J Gastroenterol. 2011;46:1230–7.

22. Yang S, Zhu H, Li Y, Lin H, Gabrielson K, Trush MA, et al. Mitochondrial adaptations to obesity-related oxidant stress. Arch Biochem Biophys. 2000;378:259–68.

23. Harrison SA. Liver disease in patients with diabetes mellitus. J Clin Gastroenterol. 2006;40:68–76.

24. Calle EE, Kaaks R. Overweight obesity and cancer: epidemiological evidence and proposed mechanisms. Nat Rev Cancer. 2004;4:579–91.

25. Hassan MM, Curley SA, Li D, et al. Association of diabetes duration and diabetes treatment with the risk of hepatocellular carcinoma. Cancer. 2010;116:1938–46.

Chapter 7
Diabetes, Specific Hepatobiliary Diseases, and Treatment

Michael Lin and S. Chris Pappas

7.1 Diabetes and Hepatitis C

There is an increased prevalence of diabetes mellitus in the hepatitis C (HCV)-infected population [1, 2]. In a cross-sectional national survey, persons 40 years of age or older with HCV infection were more than three times more likely to have type 2 diabetes than those without HCV [2]. Given the epidemiologic evidence, there has been a speculation as to whether HCV itself plays a more direct role in the development of diabetes. In a retrospective study involving over 1,100 patients, diabetes was seen in 21 % of HCV-infected patients, compared with only 12 % of noninfected patients [3]. This study suggests that the diabetes is related specifically to HCV infection, as opposed to liver disease in general. Additionally, patients who underwent liver transplantation were far more likely to develop posttransplantation diabetes if the cause of liver disease was related to HCV [4], further suggesting that HCV is directly involved in the pathogenesis of diabetes. The relationship between HCV and diabetes has

M. Lin (✉) • S.C. Pappas
Ben Taub General Hospital,
5th Fl (5-PO 71 002b) 1504 Taub Loop, Houston, TX 77030, USA
e-mail: ml4@bcm.edu; scpappas@bcm.edu

J. Sellin (ed.), *Managing Gastrointestinal Complications of Diabetes*, DOI 10.1007/978-3-319-48662-8_7,
© Springer International Publishing AG 2017

been studied closely, and there are three distinct processes that have been described [1]. First, insulin resistance and diabetes may simply be a result of progressive fibrosis caused by chronic HCV infection. Second, chronic HCV results in increasing hepatic steatosis, which leads to the development of insulin resistance. Third, chronic HCV may have a direct cytopathic effect on insulin sensitivity. Specifically, Masini and colleagues showed the presence of HCV-positive islet cells in patients with chronic HCV infection. These islet cells demonstrated certain morphological changes as well as reduced in vitro glucose-stimulated insulin release [5]. Thus, insulin resistance and diabetes may occur as a result of various direct viral or host-dependent pathways working independently or synergistically.

HCV has been shown to induce insulin resistance irrespective of the severity of liver disease [6]. The homeostatic model assessment-estimated insulin resistance (HOMA-IR) was found to be an independent predictor for the degree of fibrosis and rate of fibrosis progression in patients with HCV. The finding that insulin resistance and diabetes are important determinants of fibrosis has been demonstrated in other studies as well. The prevalence of advanced fibrosis increases progressively from patients with normal insulin sensitivity (15.8 %) to patients with insulin resistance without diabetes (29.9 %) and to patients with diabetes (58.7 %) [7]. Furthermore, the presence of diabetes negatively affects the prognosis of patients affected by HCV [8]. Diabetes was shown to be a risk factor for progression of liver fibrosis. Patients with chronic HCV and diabetes have lower cirrhosis-free survival rates, reduced time to the development of hepatocellular carcinoma, and reduced time to liver-related death.

The treatment of HCV with interferon-based therapy is impaired in the setting of diabetes [9–11]. A meta-analysis showed higher rates of sustained virologic response in patients with HCV, without evidence of insulin resistance, treated with interferon-based therapy, compared with patients with evidence of insulin resistance, irrespective of genotype

[11]. Odds ratios (ORs) for genotypes 1, 2+3, and 4 were 2.16 (95 % confidence interval [CI], 1.51–3.08), 3.06 (95 % CI, 1.06–8.82), and 6.65 (95 % CI, 2.51–17.61), respectively. At the time of publication, it remains unclear if insulin resistance and diabetes affect SVR in patients treated with direct-acting antivirals, and further investigation is needed [12].

Fortunately, the treatment of HCV infection has been shown to have a favorable effect on diabetes and insulin resistance. In fact, after 4 weeks of treatment with interferon, there may be some improvement in glucose tolerance [13]. Furthermore, patients who are able to achieve SVR have improved insulin resistance [14, 15], beta-cell function [14], and insulin hypersecretion [15]. Even in nondiabetic patients, achieving SVR prevents de novo insulin resistance [16]. Perhaps most importantly, SVR is associated with improved macrovascular and microvascular complications of diabetes including cardiovascular and renal events [17, 18]. In a study involving over 36,000 patients, the 8-year cumulative incidences of end-stage renal disease, acute coronary syndrome, and ischemic strokes between treated and untreated HCV patients were 0.15 % vs. 1.32 % ($P<0.001$), 2.21 % vs. 2.96 % ($P = 0.027$), and 1.31 % vs. 1.76 % ($P = 0.001$) [17]. These observations support the hypothesis that HCV infection may have a direct cytopathic effect on insulin sensitivity.

7.2 Diabetes and Acute Liver Failure

Acute liver failure is a rare entity with only 2,000 cases in the USA per year [19]. However, diabetes seems to increase the risk of acute liver failure [20]. The cumulative incidence of acute liver failure was significantly higher among patients with diabetes with incidence rate of 2.31 per 10,000 person-years vs. 1.44 per 10,000 person-years in the nondiabetic group. After controlling for comorbidity index, age, sex, ethnicity, and period of service, diabetes was associated with a relative risk (RR) of 1.44 (95 % CI, 1.26–1.63) for acute liver failure.

7.2.1   Hemochromatosis

No discussion of diabetes and liver disease would be complete without mention of hereditary hemochromatosis (HHC). While not primarily a liver disease, HHC affects the liver and can lead to cirrhosis, while deposition of iron in the pancreas can lead to diabetes [21]. Fortunately, the presentation of HHC with "bronze diabetes" is no longer commonly seen in clinical practice because HHC is generally diagnosed and treated before significant pancreatic islet injury has occurred. The most common presentation now is fatigue, arthralgia, and hepatomegaly [21]. Nonetheless, a general practice rule is to always consider the diagnosis of HHC when evaluating a patient with cirrhosis and diabetes. In addition, it is important to note that less frequent forms of HHC, related to *TfR2, HJV, or HAMP* gene mutations (as opposed to the more common *HFE* gene mutations), commonly present at an early age as juvenile or early-onset HHC, with diabetes and liver disease at the time of diagnosis [21].

7.3   Diabetes and Biliary Tract Disease

7.3.1   Gallstone Disease

Patients with diabetes have an increased risk of gallstone disease, which includes gallstones, cholecystitis, or gallbladder cancer; the magnitude of the increased risk has varied across studies [22]. This is possibly related to the different populations that have been evaluated and, in North America, the inclusion of patient populations known to have an increased risk of coincident diabetes and gallstone disease (e.g., Pima Indians and Mexican-Americans in the USA) [23]. A recent systematic review and meta-analysis of studies evaluating the risk of gallstone disease estimated that a diagnosis of diabetes appears to increase the relative risk of gallstone disease by 56 % [22]. Intuitively, it would seem reasonable to attribute this to common risk factors for diabetes and gallstone disease (e.g., obesity, hyperlipidemia). However, adjustment for body mass index (BMI) in a number of studies included in the meta-analysis indicated diabetes had an independent effect on the risk of gallstone disease; it has been speculated that this is related to impaired gallbladder motility as part of diabetes-related visceral neuropathy [22]. To further complicate matters, moderate to severe nonalcoholic fatty liver disease (NAFLD), commonly associated with diabetes and sharing risk factors for gallstone disease, may be associated with gallstone disease independent of risk factors for NAFLD [24].

Recognizing the increased risk of gallstones in patients with diabetes and the evidence that type 2 diabetes may be associated with an increased risk of various cancers, the risk of gallbladder cancer is of particular interest. A systematic review and meta-analysis suggests that both men and women with type 2 diabetes have an increased risk of gallbladder cancer (summary RR = 1.56, 95 % CI, 1.36–1.79), independent of smoking, BMI, and a history of gallstones [25]. The potential role of alcohol as a confounder in this study is unclear; the summary relative risk of gallbladder cancer was attenuated, but still statistically significant, when restricting the meta-analysis to studies that controlled alcohol use. While the relative risk of gallbladder cancer is increased in patients with type 2 diabetes, the absolute risk remains low (based on an overall worldwide incidence), varying from approximately 1.5 per 100,000 in North America to 25 per 100,000 in South America and Northern India [26].

Historically, the management of gallstone disease in patients with diabetes has included screening for gallstone disease and prophylactic cholecystectomy, based on the perception that patients with diabetes were at higher risk of morbidity and mortality related to the acute management of cholecystitis. However, by the early 1990s, accumulated experience and data suggested that this approach was not necessary; while the rates of operative morbidity and mortality for biliary surgery in patients with diabetes were slightly higher when compared to the general population, the rates did not rise to the level that would justify prophylactic cholecystectomy [27]. Particularly as result of the advance of laparoscopic techniques for cholecystectomy [28], current standards of care recommend that prophylactic cholecystectomy is not of benefit and should not be routinely recommended for patients with diabetes with asymptomatic gallstones; the management of gallstones in patients with diabetes is the same as that for patients without diabetes. It should be noted, however, that patients with diabetes undergoing laparoscopic cholecystectomy may require a conversion to open cholecystectomy more frequently than nondiabetic patients (independent of obesity) and may experience more postoperative complications, particularly in the setting of diabetes-related renal insufficiency [29].

7.4   Autoimmune Biliary Disease and Diabetes

Not surprisingly, autoimmune-based liver disease involving the biliary tree (i.e., primary biliary cirrhosis [PBC] and primary sclerosing cholangitis [PSC]) has been described in patients with type 1 diabetes. While a reference is occasionally made to an "association" of primary biliary cirrhosis with type 1 diabetes, most reports are individual cases [30]. It is of interest that the risk of PBC and its progression is associated with a genetic variant in a region of the cytotoxic T lymphocyte-associated antigen 4 (CTLA4) gene [31]. The risk of type 1 diabetes has also been associated with variations in this gene [32].

In contrast to PBC, the evidence for an association of PSC with type 1 diabetes, and possibly type 2, is stronger. The prevalence of type 1 diabetes in patients with PSC is 4 %, and the RR of type 1 diabetes in patients with PSC was 7.95 in a large patient cohort ($n = 678$) [33, 34]. In the latter study, the RR of type 2 was 2.54; compared with type 1, this association may be confounded by detection bias and the use of diabetogenic interventions for the treatment of PSC (e.g., high-dose steroids and immunosuppressive agents such as tacrolimus and cyclosporine A) [35].

7.5 Treatment of Coexisting Diabetes and Liver Disease

There is a strong relationship between diabetes and hepatobiliary diseases, and thus treating diabetes is important to improve outcomes for liver disease (e.g., increased cirrhosis-free survival rates, decreased frequency of hepatocellular carcinoma, and decreased liver-related death).

While still somewhat controversial, it is generally believed that chronic liver disease and cirrhosis do not increase a patient's risk of drug-induced liver injury (DILI) although these patients may be at higher risk for more complicated courses and adverse outcomes [36]. The drugs commonly used to treat diabetes rarely result in hepatotoxicity (Table 7.1) or acute liver failure (Table 7.2). Unfortunately, this was not always the case as we recall our experiences with troglitazone [37].

Troglitazone was an oral hypoglycemic medication which generated over $2 billion in sales in the late 1990s. However, it caused at least 90 cases of acute liver failure, 70 of which resulted in death or liver transplantation. After 3 years on the market, it was withdrawn. Fortunately, other thiazolidinediones (TZDs) including pioglitazone and rosiglitazone do not seem to have the same propensity for liver failure and remain available for use. Even when patients present with advanced liver disease or cirrhosis, diabetic medications are not contraindicated. However, given certain changes in physiology or metabolism, medications should be dosed cautiously (Table 7.1). For example, sulfonylureas may not be able to overcome insulin resistance and defects in insulin secretion seen in patients with cirrhosis from alcohol abuse [38–40]; therefore, a different medication should be selected in this situation.

There are instances where steroids are necessary to treat autoimmune hepatobiliary disease despite the presence of diabetes. For example, steroids are frequently necessary for achieving remission in active autoimmune hepatitis despite comorbid diabetes. Control of glucocorticoid-induced hyperglycemia is important as even short-term hyperglycemia is

Table 7.1 Antidiabetic medications and related hepatotoxicity

Drug class	Medication	Hepatotoxicity	Safe in patients with cirrhosis?	Comment
Sulfonylureas[a]	Glyburide, glipizide	Rare cholestasis	Yes	May not overcome insulin resistance and defect in insulin secretion seen in alcoholic cirrhosis
Biguanides	Metformin	None	Yes	FDA warning against the use with alcohol binge drinkers given the risk of lactic acidosis
Thiazolidinediones	Pioglitazone, rosiglitazone	Transient ALT elevation, rarely hepatitis	Yes	Available TZDs are safe and have lower risk of acute liver failure vs. troglitazone
Alpha-glucosidase inhibitors	Acarbose	Transient ALT elevation, rarely severe liver disease	Yes	
	Miglitol	None	Yes	
Meglitinides	repaglinide, nateglinide	None	Yes	
Insulin		None	Yes	May need decreased doses with decompensated liver disease due to decreased breakdown of insulin and decreased gluconeogenesis

[a]Most commonly associated with hepatotoxicity compared to any other class of antihyperglycemic medication [38–40]

TABLE 7.2 Diabetic medications and acute liver failure [38]

Drug	Prescriptions (×10⁶)	Hepatitis cases per 10⁶ prescriptions	Acute liver failure cases per 10⁵ prescriptions
Troglitazone	4.5	21.5	4.6
Rosiglitazone	4.4	14.7	0.9
Pioglitazone	3.6	9.4	0.8
Metformin	6.5	2.9	0.2
Glyburide	3.6	4.1	0

associated with elevated inflammatory markers and endothelial dysfunction in patients with and without diabetes [41, 42], as well as an increased risk of cardiovascular complications [41, 43]. When possible, patients should be treated with budesonide instead of prednisone to minimize systemic effects. In non-cirrhotic patients, budesonide undergoes significant first-pass metabolism [44, 45], thereby reducing the risk of systemic steroid toxicity [44, 46]. In cirrhotic patients, budesonide is contraindicated due to portal systemic shunting and abnormal hepatic metabolism [44, 47]. These changes result in attenuated first-pass extraction, reduced therapeutic efficacy, and systemic steroid side effects.

When steroids must be used in the setting of diabetes, the dose and duration of steroids should be minimized. Patients also need to optimize glycemic control through adjustments or additions to their medications. In patients without cirrhosis, sulfonylureas, metformin, TZDs, and insulin have been used [41]. These would also be reasonable in cirrhotic patients with the caveats discussed previously. If the decision has been made to use insulin, neutral protamine Hagedorn (NPH) insulin is often a good choice given the similarities in pharmacodynamics profile between NPH and prednisone/prednisolone.

Although the relationship may not be intuitive, diabetes is intimately connected with a variety of hepatobiliary conditions including chronic HCV, acute liver failure, hemochromatosis, and diseases of the biliary tract. Diabetes is often associated with more frequent adverse outcomes and should be managed aggressively. Fortunately, even in the setting of advanced cirrhosis, our usual armamentarium of diabetic medications can be used safely and effectively.

References

1. Harrison SA. Liver disease in patients with diabetes mellitus. J Clin Gastroenterol. 2006;40:68–76.
2. Mehta SH, Brancati FL, Sulkowski MS, Strathdee SA, Szklo M, Thomas DL. Prevalence of type 2 diabetes mellitus among persons with hepatitis C virus infection in the United States. Ann Intern Med. 2000;133:592–9.
3. Mason AL, Lau JY, Hoang N, Qian K, Alexander GJ, Xu L, et al. Association of diabetes mellitus and chronic hepatitis C virus infection. Hepatology. 1999;29:328–33.
4. Knobler H, Stagnaro-Green A, Wallenstein S, Schwartz M, Roman SH. Higher incidence of diabetes in liver transplant recipients with hepatitis C. J Clin Gastroenterol. 1998;26:30–3.
5. asini M M, Campani D, Boggi U, enicagli M M, Funel N, Pollera M, et al. Hepatitis C virus infection and human pancreatic B-cell dysfunction. Diabetes Care. 2005;28:940–1.
6. Hui JM, Archana S, Farrell GC, Bandara P, Byth K, JG K, et al. Insulin resistance is associated with chronic hepatitis C and virus infection fibrosis progression. Gastroenterology. 2003;125:1695–704.
7. Petta S, amma C C, Marco VD, Alessi N, Cabibi D, Caldarella R, et al. Insulin resistance and diabetes increases fibrosis in the liver of patients with genotype 1 HCV infection. Am J Gastroenterol. 2008;103:1136–44.
8. Kita Y, Mizukoshi E, akamura T T, Sakurai M, Takata Y, Arai K, et al. Impact of diabetes mellitus on prognosis of patients infected with hepatitis C virus. Metabolism. 2007;56:1682–8.
9. Elgouhari HM, Zein CO, Hanouneh I, Feldstein AE, Zein NN. Diabetes mellitus is associated with impaired response to antiviral therapy in chronic hepatitis C infection. Dig Dis Sci. 2009;54:2699–705.
10. Romero-Gomez M, Mar Viloria, RJ A, Salmeron J, Diago M, CM F-R, et al. Insulin resistance impairs sustained response rate to peginterferon plus ribavirin in chronic hepatitis C patients. Gastroenterology. 2005;128:636–41.

11. Eslam M, Aparcero R, Kawaguchi T, Campo JA, Sata M, Khattab MA, et al. Meta-analysis: insulin resistance and sustained virologic response in hepatitis C. Aliment Pharmacol Ther. 2011;34:297–305.

12. Boccaccio V, Bruno S. Optimal management of patients with chronic hepatitis C and comorbidities. Liver Int. 2015;35(Suppl 1):35–43.

13. Tanaka H, Shiota G, Kawasaki H. Changes in glucose tolerance after interferon-alpha therapy in patients with chronic hepatitis C. J Med. 1997;28:335–46.

14. Kawaguchi T, Ide T, Taniguchi E, Hirano E, Itou M, umie S S, et al. Clearance of HCV improves insulin resistance, beta-cell function, and hepatic expression of insulin receptor substrate 1 and 2. Am J Gastroenterol. 2007;102:570–6.

15. Kawaguchi Y, Mizuta T, Oza N, Takahashi H, Ario K, Yoshimura T, et al. Eradication of hepatitis C virus by interferon improves whole-body insulin resistance and hyperinsulinaemia in patients with chronic hepatitis C. Liver Int. 2009;29:871–7.

16. ghemo A A, Prati GM, Rumi MG, Soffredini R, D'Ambrosio R, Orsi E, et al. Sustained virologic response prevents the development of insulin resistance in patients with chronic hepatitis C. Hepatology. 2012;56:1681–7.

17. Hsu YC, Ho HJ, Huang YT, Wang HH, Wu MS, Lin JT, et al. Association between antiviral treatment and extrahepatic outcomes in patients with hepatitis C virus infection. Gut. 2015;64:495–503.

18. Hsu YC, Lin JT, Ho HJ, Kao YH, Huang YT, Hsiao NW, et al. Antiviral treatment for hepatitis C virus infection is associated with improved renal and cardiovascular outcomes in diabetic patients. Hepatology. 2014;59:1293–302.

19. Lee WM. Acute liver failure. Semin Respir Crit Care Med. 2012;33:36–45.

20. El-Serag HB, Everhart JE. Diabetes increases the risk of acute hepatic failure. Gastroenterology. 2002;122:1822–8.

21. Pietrangelo A. Hereditary hemochromatosis: pathogenesis, diagnosis, and treatment. Gastroenterology. 2010;139:393–408.

22. Aune D, Vatten LJ. Diabetes mellitus and the risk of gallbladder disease: a systematic review and meta-analysis of prospective studies. J Diabetes Complications. 2016;30:368–73.

23. Hanis CL, Ferrell RE, Tulloch BR, Schull WJ. Gallbladder disease epidemiology in Mexican Americans in Starr County. Texas Am J Epidemiol. 1985;122:820–9.

24. Lee YC, Wu JS, Yang YC, Chang CS, Lu FH, Chang CJ. Moderate to severe, but not mild, nonalcoholic fatty liver disease is associated

with increased risk of gallstone disease. Scand J Gastroenterol. 2014;49:1001–6.

25. Gu J, Yan S, Wang B, Shen F, Cao H, Fan J, Wang Y. Type 2 diabetes mellitus and risk of gallbladder cancer: a systematic review and meta-analysis of observational studies. Diabetes Metab Res Rev. 2016;32:63–72.

26. Hundal R, EA S. Gallbladder cancer: epidemiology and outcome. Clin Epidemiol. 2014;6:99–109.

27. Aucott JN, Cooper GS, Bloom AD, Aron DC. Management of gallstones in diabetic patients. Arch Intern Med. 1993;153:1053–8.

28. Udekwu PO, Sullivan WG. Contemporary experience with cholecystectomy: establishing 'benchmarks' two decades after the introduction of laparoscopic cholecystectomy. Am Surg. 2013;79:1253–7.

29. Paajanen H, uuronen S S, Nordstrom P, Miettinen P, Niskanen L. Laparoscopic versus open cholecystectomy in diabetic patients and postoperative outcome. Surg Endosc. 2011;25:764–70.

30. Ko GT, Szeto CC, Yeung VT, Chow CC, Chan H, Cockram CS. Autoimmune polyglandular syndrome and primary biliary cirrhosis. Br J Clin Pract. 1996;50:344–6.

31. Juran BD, Atkinson EJ, Schlicht EM, Fridley BL, Lazaridis KN. Primary biliary cirrhosis is associated with a genetic variant in the 3'flanking region of the CTLA4 Gene. Gastroenterology. 2008;135:1200–6.

32. Anjos SM, Tessier MC, Polychronakos C. Association of the cytotoxic T lymphocyte-associated antigen 4 gene with type 1 diabetes: evidence for independent effects of two polymorphisms on the same haplotype block. J Clin Endocrinol Metab. 2004;89:6257–65.

33. Lamberts LE, Janse M, Haagsma EB, Berg AP, Weersma RK. Immune mediated diseases in primary sclerosing cholangitis. Dig Liver Dis. 2011;43:802–6.

34. Ludvigsson JF, Bergquist A, Montgomery SM, Bahmanyar S. Risk of diabetes and cardiovascular disease in patients with primary sclerosing cholangitis. J Hepatol. 2014;60:802–8.

35. Ehlken H, Schramm C. PSC: novel disease associations providing pathogenetic clues? J Hepatol. 2014;60:687–8.

36. Chalasani N, Bjornsson E. Risk factors for idiosyncratic drug-induced liver injury. Gastroenterology. 2010;138:2246–59.

37. Gale EA. Lessons from the glitazones: a story of drug development. Lancet. 2001;357:1870–5.

38. Tolman KG, Fonseca V, Tan MH, Dalpiaz A. Narrative review: hepatobiliary disease in type 2 diabetes mellitus. Ann Intern Med. 2004;141:946–56.
39. Tolman KG, Fonseca V, Dalpiaz A, Tan MH. Spectrum of liver disease in type 2 diabetes and management of patients with diabetes and liver disease. Diabetes Care. 2007;30:734–43.
40. Garcia-Compean D, Jaquez-Quintana JO, Lavalle-Gonzalez FJ, Gonzalez-Gonzalez JA, Munoz-Espinosa LE, Villarreal-Perez JZ, et al. Subclinical abnormal glucose tolerance is a predictor of death in liver cirrhosis. World J Gastroenterol. 2014;20:7011–8.
41. Kwon S, Hermayer KL. Glucocorticoid-induced hyperglycemia. Am J Med Sci. 2013;345:274–7.
42. Ceriello A, Esposito K, Piconi L, Ihnat MA, Thorpe JE, Testa R, et al. Oscillating glucose is more deleterious to endothelial function and oxidative stress than mean glucose in normal and type 2 diabetic patients. Diabetes. 2008;57:1349–54.
43. Strohmayer E, Krakoff L. Glucocorticoids and cardiovascular risk factors. Endocrinol Metab Clin North Am. 2011;40:409–17.
44. Vierling JM. Autoimmune hepatitis and overlap syndromes: diagnosis and management. Clin Gastroenterol Hepatol. 2015;13:2088–108.
45. AJ C. Drug choices in autoimmune hepatitis: part A—steroids. Expert Rev Gastroenterol Hepatol. 2012;6:603–15.
46. Strassburg CP. Therapeutic options to treat autoimmune hepatitis in 2009. Dig Dis. 2010;28:93–8.
47. Geier A, Gartung C, Dietrich CG, Wasmuth HE, Reinartz P, Matem S. Side effects of budesonide in liver cirrhosis due to chronic autoimmune hepatitis: influence of hepatic metabolism versus portosystemic shunts on a patient complicated with HCC. World J Gastroenterol. 2003;9:2681–5.

Chapter 8
Diabetes, Cirrhosis, and Liver Transplantation

Michael Lin and S. Chris Pappas

8.1 Diabetes and Cirrhosis

In recent years, the relationship between diabetes and cirrhosis, distinct from nonalcoholic liver fatty liver disease (NAFLD), has become increasingly recognized. In addition, a significant amount of experience with diabetes in the setting of liver transplantation has accumulated. In this chapter, we will examine the relationship between diabetes and cirrhosis and provide an overview of diabetes in the liver transplantation setting.

Impaired glucose tolerance is seen in 60 % of patients with cirrhosis [1]. Overt diabetes is seen in 20 % of patients with cirrhosis. However, it is important to note that there are two distinct types of diabetes seen with chronic liver disease. Patients can either have preexisting diabetes and later go on to develop progressive liver disease or develop diabetes as a result of cirrhosis. The latter is an entity which is sometimes referred to as "hepatogenous" diabetes. Compared with those who have traditional type 2 diabetes, patients with

M. Lin • S.C. Pappas, MD, JD, FCLM, FAASLD (✉)
Ben Taub General Hospital, 5th Fl (5-PO 71 002b) 1504 Taub Loop, Houston, TX 77030, USA
e-mail: scpappas@bcm.edu

J. Sellin (ed.), *Managing Gastrointestinal Complications of Diabetes*, DOI 10.1007/978-3-319-48662-8_8,
© Springer International Publishing AG 2017

hepatogenous diabetes frequently do not have a strong family history of diabetes [2]. Furthermore, while these patients seem to have a higher degree of insulin resistance, they also seem to be at decreased risk for cardiovascular and ophthalmologic complications. These features of hepatogenous diabetes support the contention that this type of diabetes represents a clinically relevant diabetes type separate from type 1, type 2, gestational, and other types of diabetes (e.g., autoimmune diabetes). Distinguishing between preexisting diabetes with the subsequent development of coincidental liver disease and hepatogenous diabetes can be very difficult but should be attempted in view of the possible clinical implications; a careful review of family history and the time course for the development of diabetes in a patient with chronic liver disease is very important.

Multiple studies demonstrate the negative impact of diabetes on chronic liver disease and cirrhosis. Individuals with chronic liver disease and diabetes were hospitalized at a rate four times higher than those without diabetes [3]. Additionally, in a study where 53 % of cirrhotic patients were readmitted within 3 months, having a higher Model for End-Stage Liver Disease (MELD) score, the presence of diabetes, use of prophylactic antibiotics for spontaneous bacterial peritonitis (SBP), and prior hepatic encephalopathy were associated with readmission [4]. Readmitted patients had a higher prevalence of diabetes, compared to patients not readmitted (40 % vs. 33 %, $P = 0.03$); a predictive logistic regression model for readmissions showed that patients with diabetes on admission were more likely to be readmitted compared to patients without diabetes (odds ratio [OR] 1.36, 95 % confidence interval [CI], 0.98–1.88; $P = 0.07$). A recently published registry study from the UK also demonstrated that patients with diabetes were more likely to be hospitalized with a chronic liver disease than nondiabetic patients [5]. In fact, type 2 diabetes was associated with an increased incidence of hospitalizations with alcoholic liver disease (RR 1.38 in men, RR 1.57 in women), nonalcoholic fatty liver disease (RR 3.03 in men, RR 5.11 in women), autoimmune liver disease

(RR 1.50 in men, RR 1.25 in women), hemochromatosis (RR 1.67 in men, RR 1.60 in women), and hepatocellular carcinoma (RR 3.36 in men, RR 3.55 in women) [5, 6].

Diabetes has also been shown to affect liver disease complications. Diabetes is associated with events of hepatic decompensation such as development of ascites [7], variceal bleeding [8], and hepatic encephalopathy [9]. There have also been multiple studies clearly showing increased risk of hepatocellular carcinoma (HCC) in the setting of diabetes [10–12], as well as increased mortality from HCC [13]. The relationship between HCC and diabetes is discussed in more detail in Chap. 6.

Cirrhosis is an important but under-recognized cause of mortality among patients with diabetes. In a population-based study involving nearly 7,200 patients that investigated the causes of death in patients with type 2 diabetes, chronic liver disease, and cirrhosis accounted for 4.4 % [14]. The highest standardized mortality ratio (SMR) was for cirrhosis, which had an SMR of 2.52 (95 % CI, 1.96–3.20). This was even higher than the SMR for cardiovascular disease of 1.34 (95 % CI, 1.23–1.44). Additionally, diabetes has also been shown to be a risk factor affecting long-term survival in cirrhosis in multiple studies [15, 16]. Subclinical abnormal glucose tolerance has been associated with lower survival in cirrhosis [17]. However, it remains to be seen whether improvement in glycemic control results in decrease mortality in this population.

8.2   Diabetes and Liver Transplantation

Diabetes related to liver transplantation can occur either as preexisting diabetes or as new-onset posttransplantation diabetes mellitus (PTDM). Every year, there are approximately 6,000 deceased donor liver transplants and 300 living donor liver transplants in the USA alone. From 2003 to 2012, there were over 38,000 liver transplantations [18]. Of these, nearly 9,900 recipients (25.7 %) carried a diagnosis of diabetes. As liver transplant recipients are surviving longer, metabolic disorders are being seen with increasing frequency, including PTDM. The reported incidence of PTDM varies greatly, ranging from 4 % to over 30 % [2, 19]. The vast majority of PTDM are diagnosed within the first 3 months of liver transplantation [2]. The etiology of PTDM is multifactorial. Pretransplant diabetes, alcoholic cirrhosis, hepatitis C, male gender, and immunosuppressive medication including cyclosporine, tacrolimus, and corticosteroids are associated with PTDM [2].

Both preexisting diabetes and posttransplantation diabetes impact a patient's clinical course. In patients with preexisting diabetes, older studies have suggested that diabetes was not associated with a decrease in survival after liver transplantation [20, 21]. However, there are multiple, more recent studies showing a decreased survival in this population. In one case-control study involving 57 patients with preexisting diabetes and 114 age-, sex-, and race-matched patients without diabetes, survival at 1 year (87 % vs. 77 %) and 2 years (81.6 % vs. 70.1 %) was similar. However, 5-year survival was lower among patients with diabetes (34.4 % vs. 67.7 %) [22]. In a population-based study which examined all adult liver transplant recipients from 2003 to 2012 in the USA, diabetes negatively impacted survival at 5 years regardless of the presence of obesity [18]. Diabetes was found to be an independent predictor of decreased survival following liver transplantation (HR 1.29; 95 % CI, 1.21–1.36). Preexisting diabetes is also associated with increased frequency of rejection and posttransplantation complications including cardiovascular, infectious, ophthalmologic, neurologic, hematologic, and respiratory complications [22]. Graft survival appears unaffected by preexisting diabetes in the recipient; however, one study found that the presence of donor diabetes was a strong predictor of graft failure (HR 1.20) if recipients were also HCV positive [23].

The effect of PTDM on survival is less clear. In a retrospective study of 778 patients (284 with sustained PTDM, 227 without diabetes at any time) followed for a median of

57.2 months, sustained PTDM was associated with worse patient survival seemingly related to higher infection rates [24]. In a case-control trial involving 46 patients with PTDM with 92 age- and sex-matched patients without preexisting diabetes or PTDM, patient survival at 1 year (93.5 % vs. 83.5 %), 2 years (88.1 % vs. 77.9 %), and 5 years (75 % vs. 77.2 %) were similar [25]. There is also conflicting evidence on the effect of PTDM on graft survival [22, 24]. PTDM is associated with higher frequency of rejection and postoperative complications such as infection and neurologic, cardiovascular, and neuropsychiatric complications (i.e., depression).

Living donor liver transplantation (LDLT) is becoming an increasingly frequent practice given the lack of deceased donors. The literature examining LDLT and diabetes is limited. It appears that PTDM occurs less frequently after LDLT [26]. Yadav et al. examined 902 nondiabetic LDLT recipients and 19,582 nondiabetic deceased donor liver transplantation (DDLT) recipients [27]. The incidence of new-onset PTDM after LDLT was 7.4 %, 2.1 %, and 2.6 % at 1, 3, and 5 years, respectively, compared with the incidences of 12.5 %, 3.4 %, and 1.9 % at 1, 3, and 5 years, respectively, after DDLT. Risk factors for developing PTDM after LDLT include hepatitis C, treated acute cellular rejection, older age of the recipient, and hypertriglyceridemia [26, 28]. Either way, PTDM did not affect patient morbidity and mortality [28].

Our understanding of PTDM is constantly evolving. Wilkinson et al. have proposed a practical treatment and management guideline for PTDM (Fig. 8.1) [29]. Prior to liver transplantation, transplant candidates should be monitored for impaired glucose tolerance and diabetes through some combination of fasting plasma glucose, oral glucose tolerance testing, or hemoglobin A1c check. When appropriate, patients should receive counseling on weight control, diet, and exercise. To reduce diabetogenic risk, early corticosteroid dose reduction and minimization or discontinuation of calcineurin inhibitors should be considered. After liver

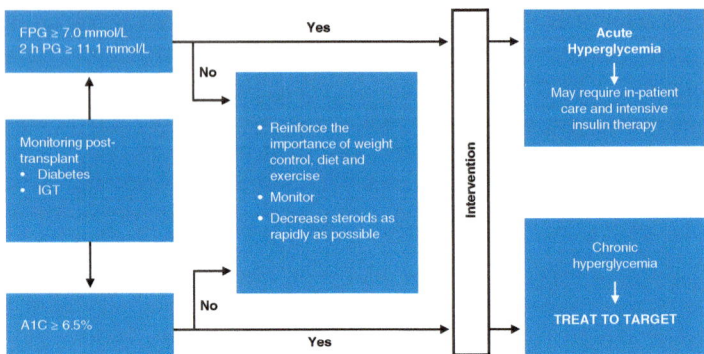

FIGURE 8.1 Posttransplant management: blood glucose control. *FPG* fasting plasma glucose, *IGT* impaired glucose tolerance, *PG* plasma glucose (Reproduced with permission from Wilkinson [29] ©Wiley)

transplantation, all patients should be closely monitored for PTDM. Patients with acute hyperglycemia with blood glucose level above 360 mg/dL should receive immediate intervention. Management of chronic hyperglycemia or PTDM should follow guidelines from the American Diabetes Association and/or other major consensus guidelines [30].

References

1. Tolman KG, Fonseca V, Dalpiaz A, Tan MH. Spectrum of liver disease in type 2 diabetes and management of patients with diabetes and liver disease. Diabetes Care. 2007;30:734–43.
2. Harrison SA. Liver disease in patients with diabetes mellitus. J Clin Gastroenterol. 2006;40:68–76.
3. Byrd KK, Mehal JM, Schillie SF, Holman RC, Haberling D, Murphy T. Chronic liver disease-associated hospitalizations among adults with diabetes, national inpatient sample, 2001–2012. Public Health Rep. 2015;130:693–703.
4. Bajaj JS, Reddy KR, Tandon P, Wong F, Kamath PS, arcia-Tsao G G, et al. The 3-month readmission rate remains unacceptably high in a large North American cohort of cirrhotic patients. Hepatology. 2016;64:200–8.

5. Wild SH, Morling JR, McAllister DA, Kerssens J, Fischbacher C, Parkes J, et al. Type 2 diabetes and risk of hospital admission or death for chronic liver disease. J Hepatol. 2016;64:1358–64.

6. Wong VW, Chalasani N. Not routine screening, but vigilance for chronic liver disease in patients with type 2 diabetes. J Hepatol. 2016;64:1211–3.

7. Elkrief L, Chouinard P, Bendesky N, Hajage D, Larroque B, Babany G, et al. Diabetes mellitus is an independent prognostic factor for major liver-related outcomes in patients with cirrhosis and chronic hepatitis C. Hepatology. 2014;60:823–31.

8. Jeon HK, Kim MY, Baik SK, Park HJ, Choi H, Park SY, et al. Hepatogenous diabetes in cirrhosis is related to portal pressure and variceal hemorrhage. Dig Dis Sci. 2013;58:3335–41.

9. Jepsen P, Watson H, PK A, Vilstrup H. Diabetes as a risk for hepatic encephalopathy in cirrhosis patients. J Hepatol. 2015;63:1133–8.

10. Hassan MM, Hwang LY, Hatten CJ, Swaim M, Li D, Abbruzzcsc JL, et al. Risk factors for hepatocellular carcinoma: synergism of alcohol with viral hepatitis and diabetes mellitus. Hepatology. 2002;36:1206–13.

11. Davila JA, Morgan RO, Shaib Y, McGlynn KA, El-Serag HB. Diabetes increases the risk of hepatocellular carcinoma in the United States: a population based case control study. Gut. 2005;54:533–9.

12. El-Serag HB, Tran T, Everhart JE. Diabetes increases the risk of chronic liver disease and hepatocellular carcinoma. Gastroenterology. 2004;126:460–8.

13. Raffetti E, Portolani N, Molfino S, Baiocchi GL, Limina RM, Caccamo G, et al. Role of aetiology, diabetes, tobacco smoking, and hypertension in hepatocellular carcinoma survival. Dig Liver Dis. 2015;47:950–6.

14. Marco R, Locatelli F, Zoppini G, Verlato G, Bonora E, uggeo M M. Cause-specific mortality in type 2 diabetes. The Verona diabetes study. Diabetes Care. 1999;22:756–61.

15. Bianchi G, Marchesini G, Zoli M, Bugianesi E, Fabbri A, Pisi E. Prognostic significance of diabetes in patients with cirrhosis. Hepatology. 1994;20:119–25.

16. Quintana JO, Garcia-Compean D, Gonzalez JA, Perez JZ, Gonzalez FJ, Espinosa LE, et al. The impact of diabetes mellitus in mortality in patients with compensated liver cirrhosis-a prospective study. Ann Hepatol. 2011;10:56–62.

17. Garcia-Compean D, Jaquez-Quintana JO, Lavalle-Gonzalez FJ, Gonzalez-Gonzalez JA, Munoz-Espinosa LE, Villarreal-Perez JZ, et al. Subclinical abnormal glucose tolerance is a predictor of death in liver cirrhosis. World J Gastroenterol. 2014;20:7011–8.

18. Wong RJ, Cheung R, Perumpail RB, Holt EW, hmed A A. Diabetes mellitus, and not obesity, is associated with lower survival following liver transplantation. Dig Dis Sci. 2015;60:1036–44.

19. Saliba F, Lakehal M, Pageaux G, Roche B, Vanlemmens C, Duvoux C, et al. Risk factors for new-onset diabetes mellitus following liver transplantation and impact of hepatitis C infection: an observational multicenter study. Liver Transpl. 2007;13:136–44.

20. Trail KC, Stratta RJ, Larsen JL, El R, Patil KD, AN L, et al. Results of liver transplantation in diabetic recipients. Surgery. 1993;114:650–6.

21. Wahlstrom HE, Cooper J, ores G G, Rosen C, Wiesner R, Krom RA. Survival after liver transplantation in diabetics. Transplant Proc. 1991;23:1565–6.

22. John PR, Thuluvath PJ. Outcome of liver transplantation in patients with diabetes mellitus: a case-control study. Hepatology. 2001;34:889–95.

23. Wu Y, hmed A A, Kamal A. Donor diabetes mellitus is an independent risk factor for graft loss in HCV positive but not HCV negative liver transplant recipients. Dig Dis Sci. 2013;58:574–8.

24. Moon JI, Barbeito R, Faradji RN, Gaynor JJ, Tzakis AG. Negative impact of new-onset diabetes mellitus on patient and graft survival after liver transplantation: long-term follow up. Transplantation. 2006;82:1625–8.

25. John PR, Thuluvath PJ. Outcome of patients with new-onset diabetes mellitus after liver transplantation compared with those without diabetes mellitus. Liver Transpl. 2002;8:708–13.

26. Kuo HT, Sampaio MS, Ye X, Reddy P, Martin P, Bunnapradist S. Risk factors for new-onset diabetes mellitus in adult liver transplant recipients, an analysis of the Organ Procurement and Transplant Network/United Network for Organ Sharing database. Transplantation. 2010;89:1134–40.

27. AD Y, Chang YH, Agel BA, Byrne TJ, HA C, Douglas DD, et al. New onset diabetes mellitus in living donor versus deceased donor liver transplant recipients: analysis of the UNOS/OPTN database. J Transplant. 2013;2013:269096.

28. Abe T, Onoe T, Tahara H, Tashiro H, Ishiyama K, Ide K, et al. Risk factors for development of new-onset diabetes mellitus and progressive impairment of glucose metabolism after living-donor liver transplantation. Transplant Proc. 2014;46:865–9.
29. Wilkinson A, Davidson J, Dotta F, Home PD, Keown P, Kiberd B, et al. Guidelines for the treatment and management of new-onset diabetes after transplantation. Clin Transplant. 2005;19:291–8.
30. Standard of Medical Care in Diabetes – 2016. Diabetes Care. 2016;39(Supplement):S1–112.

Chapter 9
Diabetes and the Exocrine Pancreas

David Tang and Robert J. Sealock

9.1 Overview of Acinar/Ductal Anatomy and Function

The working unit of the exocrine pancreas is the *acinus*, Latin for cluster of berries. Analogous to its namesake, acinar morphology consists of individual acinar cells arranged in a spherical cluster with apical regions oriented toward the center. Digestive enzymes synthesized and stored in the acinar cell are secreted across the apical membrane and prevented from passing between acinar cells by intracellular tight junctions. Clusters of acini are themselves arranged into lobules. The lumen of the acinus communicates with intralobular ducts, which empty into interlobular ducts and, in turn, drain into the main pancreatic duct. The lumen of the pancreatic ductal system is lined with the epithelium that specializes in secretion of inorganic ions, especially bicarbonate, in an endocrine signal-dependent and isotonic fashion. In this way, the acinus is primarily responsible for digestive enzyme synthesis, and the ductal epithelium is primarily responsible for inorganic ion and aqueous component of pancreatic secretions.

D. Tang • R.J. Sealock, MD (⊠)
Baylor College of Medicine, Department of Gastroenterology and Hepatology, Houston, TX, USA
e-mail: rjsealoc@bcm.edu

J. Sellin (ed.), *Managing Gastrointestinal Complications of Diabetes*, DOI 10.1007/978-3-319-48662-8_9,
© Springer International Publishing AG 2017

9.2   Endocrine Control of Pancreatic Ductal Secretion

Both acinar and ductal epithelial cell secretions are governed by endocrine and neurocrine signaling. Secretin is a small peptide produced by S cells in the small intestine in response to gastric acid. Secretin signaling results in increased bicarbonate secretion by the ductal epithelium leading to water influx into the duct to maintain isotonicity and increasing flow rate. Bicarbonate neutralization of duodenal acid then shuts off secretin production, completing the negative feedback loop.

Cholecystokinin (CCK) is produced by I cells in the small intestine in response peptides, amino acids, and fatty acids from a meal. Acinar response to CCK is achieved indirectly though neurohormonal response of the vagus nerve mediated by neuronal CCK-1 receptors, leading to increased volume of pancreatic enzymatic secretions. Gastrin is a related peptide released predominantly in the gastric antrum in response to peptides and fatty acids and gastric distention in a pH-dependent fashion and also increases pancreatic enzyme secretion via CCK-1 receptors in an analogous neurohormonal fashion as CCK.

Somatostatin is a peptide produced by D cells in the gastric and intestinal mucosa as well as by delta cells of the pancreatic islets. Somatostatin exhibits broad inhibitory actions in the gastrointestinal (GI) tract including decreasing pancreatic enzyme and fluid secretions.

9.3   Imaging the Pancreas and Measuring Pancreatic Function

Imaging of the pancreas has rapidly evolved in the past decades driven by the limitation of traditional invasive and noninvasive pancreatic imaging. Transabdominal ultrasound was one of the first methods of imaging the pancreas but does not reliably demonstrate the organ due to obscuration by intestinal gas. Multi-detector computerized tomography (CT) may demonstrate gland atrophy and calcifications but is not reliable for early chronic pancreatitis. MRI and magnetic resonance cholangiopancreatography (MRCP) are much more reliable and accurate but similarly limited in detection of early disease. Secretin-enhanced MRCP improves sensitivity to early chronic pancreatitis. Secretin stimulates pancreatic secretion while simultaneously increasing sphincter of Oddi tone acutely, therefore filling peripheral ductal branches with fluid allowing for imaging of mild changes that escape the notice of conventional MRCP [1]. Endoscopic retrograde cholangiopancreatography (ERCP) may also be more sensitive to early chronic pancreatitis but is associated with complications, and imaging is limited to the pancreatic ductal system without being able to directly assess the parenchyma [2]. ERCP is rarely performed purely for diagnosis due to these limitations.

Endoscopic ultrasound (EUS) has been established as a useful test for diagnosis of early small duct or "minimal change" chronic pancreatitis, and both parenchymal and ductal ultrasonographic features have been incorporated into the Rosemont criteria for diagnosis of chronic pancreatitis, a consensus diagnostic system (Table 9.1) [3]. A number of advanced imaging techniques, including digital image analysis and elastography, have been investigated as potential adjuncts to EUS, but these studies have so far been preliminary in scope, small in size, and predominantly focused on identification of malignancy rather than early parenchymal changes of chronic pancreatitis [4, 5].

However, even perfectly sensitive tests for chronic pancreatitis may not be diagnostic of exocrine insufficiency. Steatorrhea does not occur until the pancreas has lost 90 % of its exocrine reserve [6]. There may be significant discordance between EUS findings of chronic pancreatitis and exocrine insufficiency as measured by secretin pancreatic function testing [7, 8], implying that parenchymal changes

TABLE 9.1 Rosemont consensus diagnosis of chronic pancreatitis by
parenchymal and ductal features on endoscopic ultrasound

Major criteria	Minor criteria
Major criteria A	Cysts
Hyperechoic foci with shadowing (parenchymal calcifications)	Stranding
Main pancreatic duct calculi	Hyperechoic foci without shadowing
	Lobularity without honeycombing
Major criteria B	Irregular main pancreatic duct contour
Lobularity with honeycombing	Dilated main pancreatic duct
	Hyperechoic main pancreatic duct margin
	Dilated side branches

Consistent with chronic pancreatitis

1 major A feature (+) ≥3 minor features

1 major A feature (+) major B feature

2 major A features

Suggestive of chronic pancreatitis

1 major A feature (+) <3 minor features

1 major B feature (+) ≥3 minor features

≥5 minor features (any)

Indeterminate for chronic pancreatitis

3 to 4 minor features, no major features

1 major B feature alone or with <3 minor features

Normal

≤2 minor features (except for cysts, dilated main pancreatic
duct, hyperechoic foci without shadowing, and dilated side
branches, with no major features)

and exocrine insufficiency may occur concurrently or that there is a significant reserve capacity for absorption that is still adequate in early parenchymal disease. Instead of inferring pancreatic function from structural diagnosis via pancreatic imaging, direct and indirect tests of pancreatic function may be preferred for definitive diagnosis of pancreatic exocrine insufficiency.

Traditional secretin test of pancreatic function is performed by placing a double-lumen "Dreiling" tube under fluoroscopy so that distal port is in the duodenum and the proximal port in the stomach. After aspiration of gastric contents, duodenal secretions are stimulated by secretin or CCK and collected for bicarbonate and enzymatic content for upward of 1 h in serial increments. This test is both uncomfortable for the patient and also laborious for the lab and therefore rarely performed. Endoscopic pancreatic function testing (EPFT) maintains the same principles of Dreiling tube testing but has the advantage of improving patient tolerance and operator convenience by performing the test under sedation during EUS or routine upper endoscopy [9, 10]. However, specimen collection time remains up to 1 h. Indirect tests of pancreatic function avoid intestinal intubation and the hassle and expense of traditional function testing.

Fecal fat is not specific to pancreatic exocrine insufficiency but instead a measure of global malabsorption. Quantitative fecal fat analysis is performed after amassing a 72-h stool collection, while the patient maintains intake of 100 g of fat/day and subsequent titration to yield fecal fat per 24 h. The upper limit of normal for fat excretion in stool is considered 7 g/day on a 100 g of fat/day diet. But an otherwise healthy patient with induced diarrhea can have as much as 14 g fat in the stool per day [11]. In general, very high fecal fats (>30 gm/day) are associated with pancreatic insufficiency, whereas milder steatorrhea (10–30 gm/day) are more suggestive of mucosal disease.

Stool may also be stained and examined under microscopy in a qualitative test as a screen for fat malabsorption (Sudan stain). Acidification of the stool mixture allows for staining of both split fats (fatty acids) and neutral fats (triglycerides). The test can be performed without acidification which results in preferential staining of triglycerides. Increased staining for neutral fats implies a disorder of digestion such as pancreatic exocrine insufficiency, while increased staining for split fats implies malabsorption at the brush border.

Fecal chymotrypsin and elastase testing have the advantage of convenient testing on random stool collections but are hampered by being insensitive to mild-to-moderate pancreatic exocrine insufficiency, though they are very sensitive for severe disease causing steatorrhea. Fecal chymotrypsin activity assays are also affected by exogenous pancreatic enzyme supplementation which must be stopped beforehand. In addition, fecal elastase ELISA assays are more sensitive than fecal chymotrypsin, and the antibody test is specific for human elastase while being not affected by pancreatic enzyme supplementations. However, fecal elastase testing is also insensitive for mild-to-moderate pancreatic insufficiency. Both tests may produce false-positive results if the submitted stool sample is unformed and dilute (i.e., dilution from diarrhea) [12, 13].

The 13C-mixed triglyceride breath test measures $13CO_2$ after 13C-marked triglyceride is cleaved by lipase, absorbed by the gut, and metabolized by the liver. Exhaled breath samples are collected every 30 min for 6 h after ingestion of the marked meal. The sensitivity of the test for diagnosis of fat maldigestion is higher than 90 % but suffers from its unavailability in routine clinical practice [14].

The bentiromide, or N-benzoyl-tyrosyl para-aminobenzoic acid (NBT-PABA), test is sensitive for severe pancreatic insufficiency and malabsorption but, as with other indirect tests of pancreatic dysfunction, not sensitive to mild or moderate pancreatic impairment. Additionally, the test is hampered by being nonspecific for pancreatic exocrine dysfunction as any limitation in enterocyte absorption, liver conjugation, or renal secretion may result in false-positive results [12, 15]. In addition, the substrate necessary to perform the test is currently not available in the United States, though it is available in Europe.

Another indirect test operating on the same principles as the bentiromide test is the fluorescein dilaurate assay. It too relies on hydrolysis of the fluorescein dilaurate by specific pancreatic arylesterases to yield fluorescein, which is then absorbed and collected in the urine. This is then compared to urine fluorescein measured after free fluorescein ingestion on another day and reported as a ratio [16].

9.4   Pancreatic Exocrine Insufficiency in Diabetes

On average, 51 % of patients with type 1 diabetes mellitus and 35 % of patients with type 2 diabetes mellitus demonstrate pancreatic exocrine insufficiency (PEI) on fecal elastase testing where PEI is defined as fecal elastase less than 200 μg/g [17]. In a study of 1,000 patients with diabetes, including 697 with type 2 diabetes, 28.5 % of patients with type 1 and 19.9 % of patients with type 2 diabetes had severe PEI as defined by fecal elastase less than 100 μg/g [18]. In patients with type 2 diabetes, levels of fecal elastase may be lower in those with poor glycemic control [19]. However, there is a wide range of prevalence of PEI in these studies, with one cross-sectional study yielding only 6 % in type 1 diabetes, 10 % in patients with type 2 diabetes using insulin, and no patients with PEI and type 2 diabetes who did not require insulin [20]. The wide range of prevalence in existing studies may be due to publication bias, sampling bias (predominantly Caucasian patients sampled), reliance on a single diagnostic test of PEI (fecal elastase), as well as lack of age-matched controls of patients with other chronic conditions.

Given wide-ranging estimates, it is difficult to determine the true prevalence of PEI in patients with diabetes, especially as it translates to steatorrhea and maldigestion. Fecal elastase may be insensitive to mild and moderate pancreatic insufficiency, as well falsely positive in dilute specimens (i.e., diarrhea), and its relevance for clinical maldigestion and clinical steatorrhea remains poorly delineated in diabetic patients. Even so, there is a subset of patients with PEI as measured by fecal elastase who have clinical symptoms. In one study of patients with diabetes and abnormal fecal elastase testing, 60 % were found to have steatorrhea by quantitative fecal fat analysis, with 27 % of these patients having clinical steator- rhea [21]. Pancreatic enzyme replacement for patients with pancreatic insufficiency due to diabetes is unstudied.

Changes in gross and histological pancreatic morphology frequently accompany diabetes mellitus and may be a plau- sible link between diabetes and chronic pancreatitis. Pancreatic atrophy is often seen in autopsy studies of diabe- tes patients as well as with ultrasonography, computed tomography, and magnetic resonance imaging (MRI) [22–24]. Morphological changes of the pancreas in diabetes may be partially explained by the lack of trophic effect of insulin on acinar tissue. Residual exocrine function correlates well with residual beta-cell function in type 1 diabetes mellitus [25]. Yet, because not every patient with type 1 diabetes has pan- creatic exocrine insufficiency, trophic action of insulin must not be the only factor. Indeed, as much of the close regulation of pancreatic exocrine function is carried out by neurohor- monal mediators, diabetic neuropathy may also play a role in exocrine insufficiency in diabetics [26].

9.5   Diabetes in the Setting of Pancreatic Disease

Though the true prevalence of PEI arising from diabetes is not definitively known, PEI leading to diabetes mellitus, termed type 3c diabetes (T3cDM) [27], appears to be less common and accounts for 5–10 % of diabetic populations [28]. A T3cDM diagnosis is made in the absence of type 1 diabetes autoimmune markers and in the setting of imaging and laboratory evidence of PEI [29]. Management of T3cDM has not been well studied, given large trials have excluded this subset of patients. The conventional belief is that patients with T3cDM encounter frequent episodes of hypoglycemia due to a lack of counter-regulator hormones such as somatostatin and glucagon. In a cohort of patients with T3cDM as a result of total pancreatectomy, no patients reported a severe hypoglycemic event, and HbA1c values were not statistically different from the entire diabetic population [30]. Without dedicated clinical trials, treatment for type 3c diabetes is not standardized and commonly reflects methods used for type 2 diabetes. Given its antineoplastic and antidiabetic properties, metformin may be beneficial in this subset of patients.

9.6 Diabetes and Pancreatic Adenocarcinoma

Diabetes has been associated with an increased risk of cancer. In a Swedish population study, 24 cancer types were found to have an increased incidence among those with type 2 diabetes. Pancreatic cancer had the highest standardized incidence ratio of 2.98 (observed/expected cancer cases) compared to other cancer sites [31].

The three cell types found in the normal pancreas include acinar, ductal, and islet cells. Acinar cells comprise a majority of the organ volume (80 %), but greater than 85 % of malignant lesions arise from the ductal structures resulting in adenocarcinoma. With the increasing utilization of cross-sectional imaging, identification of premalignant lesions such as intraductal papillary mucinous neoplasm, mucinous cystic neoplasm, and solid-pseudopapillary tumors may be detected and intervened before the advent of carcinoma. This scenario remains the exception as most pancreatic cancer arises in the absence of a known premalignant lesion.

According to the Surveillance, Epidemiology, and End Results (SEER) Program, pancreatic cancer is the twelfth most common cancer and the second most common gastrointestinal type behind colorectal cancer [32]. For example, pancreatic cancer represents 3 % of all new cancer cases within the United States. Given the poor long-term survival rates, incidence and prevalence of the pancreatic cancer are similar. As with all malignancy, the rate of survival is dependent upon the stage at the time of diagnosis, with localized and metastatic pancreatic cancer survival rates of 27.1 % and 2.4 %, respectively. The unfortunate reality is a majority of those with pancreatic cancer present with metastatic disease (53 %) given the lack of symptoms at early stages. Males are affected more than females, and the median age at time of diagnosis is 71.

A variety of modifiable risk factors for pancreatic cancer have been described (Table 9.2). Tobacco use is the most recognized and understood and contributes to 35 % of pancreatic cancer cases [33]. Circulating nitrosamines and polycyclic aromatic hydrocarbons cause mutations in proto-oncogenes and tumor suppressor genes. In patients with a first episode of acute pancreatitis, smoking in combination with alcohol increases the risk of developing chronic pancreatitis (cumulative risk 30 %), a known risk factor for pancreatic cancer [34].

The presence of diabetes has also been demonstrated in >40 % of patients with a diagnosis of pancreatic cancer [35]. This is in contrast to the 15 % prevalence of diabetes within

TABLE 9.2 Modifiable risk factors of pancreatic adenocarcinoma

Risk factor	Relative risk of pancreatic carcinoma
>3 alcoholic drinks per day	1.2–1.4
Chronic pancreatitis	13.3
BMI >40 kg/m^3, male	1.5
BMI >40 kg/m^3, female	2.8
Type 1 diabetes	2.0
Type 2 diabetes	1.8
Cholecystectomy	1.2
Gastrectomy	1.5
Helicobacter pylori infection	1.4

the US population. Meta-analyses have demonstrated an increased risk of pancreatic cancer in those with diabetes(age- and sex-adjusted odds ratio 1.82) When stratified by duration of diabetes, patients with diabetes for less than 4 years had a much higher odds ratio of developing pancreatic cancer compared to those with disease duration greater than 4 years (2.1 vs. 1.5, respectively) [35]. Similarly, in a matched case/control study, the prevalence of pancreatic cancer was statically higher only in patients with a duration of diabetes of 3 years or less [35]. Given the temporal association, diabetes may be a result of pancreatic cancer as opposed to pancreatic cancer being a result of diabetes. Diabetes associated with pancreatic cancer may represent a paraneoplastic process with secreted tumor products leading to glucose intolerance and altered glucose metabolism in the liver and skeletal muscle [33].

In patients diagnosed with diabetes, is it justified to screen for pancreatic cancer? Prospective studies are lacking. Given the low prevalence of pancreatic cancer in those with newly diagnosed diabetes (1 %), a screening test must be low cost, highly sensitive, and noninvasive. These screening criteria do not currently exist. Risk-stratifying patients with newly diagnosed diabetes, a higher incidence of pancreatic cancer was found in those with lower BMI (<27), tobacco use, and parental history of pancreatic cancer [36].

In conclusion, diabetes has been associated with pancreatic cancer with risk being highest in those with diabetes for less than 3 years. Risk of pancreatic cancer does not increase as the duration of diabetes increases. Given the lack of cost-effective, noninvasive, and sensitive screening tests for pancreatic cancer, population-wide screening for pancreatic cancer in those with diabetes is prohibitive.

References

1. Sai J-K. Diagnosis of mild chronic pancreatitis (Cambridge classification): comparative study using secretin injection-magnetic resonance cholangiopancreatography and endoscopic retrograde pancreatography. World J Gastroenterol. 2008;14:1218.

2. Bozkurt T, Braun U, Leferink S, Gilly G, Lux G. Comparison of pancreatic morphology and exocrine functional impairment in patients with chronic pancreatitis. Gut. 1994;35:1132–6.
3. Catalano MF, Sahai A, Levy M, Romagnuolo J, Wiersema M, Brugge W, et al. EUS-based criteria for the diagnosis of chronic pancreatitis: the Rosemont classification. Gastrointest Endosc. 2009;69:1251–61.
4. Irisawa A, Mishra G, Hernandez LV, Bhutani MS. Quantitative analysis of endosonographic parenchymal echogenicity in patients with chronic pancreatitis. J Gastroenterol Hepatol. 2004;19:1199–205.
5. Janssen J, Schlörer E, Greiner L. EUS elastography of the pancreas: feasibility and pattern description of the normal pancreas, chronic pancreatitis, and focal pancreatic lesions. Gastrointest Endosc. 2007;65:971–8.
6. DiMagno EP, Go VL, Summerskill WH. Relations between pancreatic enzyme outputs and malabsorption in severe pancreatic insufficiency. N Engl J Med. 1973;288:813–5.
7. Stevens T. Update on the role of endoscopic ultrasound in chronic pancreatitis. Curr Gastroenterol Rep. 2011;13:117–22.
8. Conwell DL, Zuccaro G, Morrow JB, Van Lente F, Obuchowski N, Vargo JJ, et al. Cholecystokinin-stimulated peak lipase concentration in duodenal drainage fluid: a new pancreatic function test. Am J Gastroenterol. 2002;97:1392–7.
9. Conwell DL, Zuccaro G, Vargo JJ, Trolli PA, Vanlente F, Obuchowski N, et al. An endoscopic pancreatic function test with synthetic porcine secretin for the evaluation of chronic abdominal pain and suspected chronic pancreatitis. Gastrointest Endosc. 2003;57:37–40.
10. Stevens T, Conwell DL, Zuccaro G, Van Lente F, Lopez R, Purich E, Fein S. A prospective crossover study comparing secretin-stimulated endoscopic and Dreiling tube pancreatic function testing in patients evaluated for chronic pancreatitis. Gastrointest Endosc. 2008;67:458–66.
11. Fine KD, Ogunji F. A new method of quantitative fecal fat microscopy and its correlation with chemically measured fecal fat output. Am J Clin Pathol. 2000;113:528–34.
12. Chowdhury RS, Forsmark CE. Pancreatic function testing. Aliment Pharmacol Ther. 2003;17:733–50.
13. Lankisch PG. Now that fecal elastase is available in the United States, should clinicians start using it? Curr Gastroenterol Rep. 2004;6:126–31.

14. JE D–M, Iglesias–García J, Vilariño–Insua M, Iglesias–Rey M. 13C- mixed triglyceride breath test to assess oral enzyme substitution therapy in patients with chronic pancreatitis. Clin Gastroenterol Hepatol. 2007;5:484–8.

15. Glasbrenner B, Kahl S, Malfertheiner P. Modern diagnostics of chronic pancreatitis. Eur J Gastroenterol Hepatol. 2002;14:935–41.

16. Malfertheiner P, Büchler M, Müller A, Ditschuneit H. Fluorescein dilaurate serum test: a rapid tubeless pancreatic function test. Pancreas. 1987;2:53–60.

17. Hardt PD, Ewald N. Exocrine pancreatic insufficiency in diabetes mellitus: a complication of diabetic neuropathy or a different type of diabetes? Exp Diabetes Res 2011;2011:1–7.

18. Hardt PD, Hauenschild A, Nalop J, Marzeion AM, Jaeger C, Teichmann J, et al. High prevalence of exocrine pancreatic insufficiency in diabetes mellitus. Pancreatology. 2003;3:395–402.

19. Terzin V, Várkonyi T, Szabolcs A, et al. Prevalence of exocrine pancreatic insufficiency in type 2 diabetes mellitus with poor glycemic control. Pancreatology. 2014;14:356–60.

20. Vujasinovic M, Zaletel J, Tepes B, Popic B, Makuc J, Epsek Lenart M, et al. Low prevalence of exocrine pancreatic insufficiency in patients with diabetes mellitus. Pancreatology. 2013;13:343–6.

21. Hardt PD, Hauenscild A, Teichmann J, Bretzel RG, Kloer HU, S2453112/S2453113 Study Group. High prevalence of steatorrhea in 101 diabetic patients likely to suffer from exocrine pancreatic insufficiency according to low fecal elastase 1 concentrations: a prospective multicenter study. Dig Dis Sci. 2003;48:1688–92.

22. Fonseca V, Berger LA, Beckett AG, Dandona P. Size of pancreas in diabetes mellitus: a study based on ultrasound. Br Med J. 1985;291:1240–1.

23. Gilbeau JP, Poncelet V, Libon E, Derue G, Heller FR. The density, contour, and thickness of the pancreas in diabetics: CT findings in 57 patients. AJR Am J Roentgenol. 1992;159:527–31.

24. Bilgin M, Balci NC, Momtahen AJ, Bilgin Y, Klör H-U, Rau WS. MRI and MRCP findings of the pancreas in patients with diabetes mellitus. J Clin Gastroenterol. 2009;43:165–70.

25. Cavalot F, Bonomo K, Perna P, Bacillo E, Salacone P, Gallo M, et al. Pancreatic elastase-1 in stools, a marker of exocrine pancreas function, correlates with both residual-cell secretion and metabolic control in type 1 diabetic subjects. Diabetes Care. 2004;27:2052–4.

26. Newih EL H, Dooley CP, Saad C, Staples J, Zeidler A, Valenzuela JE. Impaired exocrine pancreatic function in diabetics with diarrhea and peripheral neuropathy. Dig Dis Sci. 1998;33:705–10.

27. Rickels MR, Bellin M, Toledo FGS, Robertson RP, Andersen DK, Chari ST, Brand R, Frulloni L, Anderson MA, Whitcomb DC. Detection, evaluation and treatment of diabetes mellitus in chronic pancreatitis: recommendations from pancreas fest 2012. Pancreatology. 2013;13:336–42.

28. Ewald N, Kaufmann C, Raspe A, Kloer HU, Bretzel RG, Hardt PD. Prevalence of diabetes mellitus secondary to pancreatic diseases (type 3c). Diabetes Metab Res Rev. 2012;28:338–42.

29. Ewald N, Bretzel RG. Diabetes mellitus secondary to pancreatic diseases (type 3c) — are we neglecting an important disease? Eur J Intern Med. 2013;24:203–6.

30. Jethwa P, Sodergren M, Lala A, Webber J, Buckels JAC, Bramhall SR, Mirza DF. Diabetic control after total pancreatectomy. Dig Liver Dis. 2006;38:415–9.

31. Liu X, Hemminki K, Försti A, Sundquist K, Sundquist J, Ji J. Cancer risk in patients with type 2 diabetes mellitus and their relatives. Int J Cancer. 2015;137:903–10.

32. SEER Cancer Statistics Factsheets: Pancreatic cancer. National Cancer Institute. Bethesda. http://seer.cancer.gov/statfacts/html/pancreas.html. Accessed July 25, 2016.

33. Becker AE, Hernandez YG, Frucht H, Lucas AL. Pancreatic ductal adenocarcinoma: risk factors, screening, and early detection. World J Gastroenterol. 2014;20:11182–98.

34. Ahmed Ali U, Issa Y, Hagenaars JC, Bakker OJ, van Goor H, Nieuwenhuijs VB, et al. Risk of recurrent pancreatitis and progression to chronic pancreatitis after a first episode of acute pancreatitis. Clin Gastroenterol Hepatol. 2016;14:738–46.

35. Chari ST, Leibson CL, Rabe KG, Timmons LJ, Ransom J, de Andrade M, Petersen GM. Pancreatic cancer-associated diabetes mellitus: prevalence and temporal association with diagnosis of cancer. Gastroenterology. 2008;134:95–101.

36. Huxley R, Ansary-Moghaddam A, Berrington de González A, Barzi F, Woodward M. Type-II diabetes and pancreatic cancer: a meta-analysis of 36 studies. Br J Cancer. 2005;92:2076–83.